Contemporary Masculinities

Brendan Gough

Contemporary Masculinities

Embodiment, Emotion and Wellbeing

palgrave
macmillan

Brendan Gough
Leeds Beckett University
Leeds, UK

ISBN 978-3-319-78818-0   ISBN 978-3-319-78819-7   (eBook)
https://doi.org/10.1007/978-3-319-78819-7

Library of Congress Control Number: 2018939241

Cover illustration: Pattern adapted from an Indian cotton print produced in the 19th century

Printed on acid-free paper

This Palgrave Pivot imprint is published by the registered company Springer International Publishing AG part of Springer Nature.
The registered company address is: Gewerbestrasse 11, 6330 Cham, Switzerland

For my son Finn, in my biased opinion a great exemplar of sophisticated young masculinity—but also for my daughter Darcy, a strong female who insists on nothing less from the men in the house. And for Majella, for all her support, emotional and academic, over the years—and for making me a better man.

PREFACE

I have been wanting to write a single-authored book for a while now. Previous books have mostly involved co-authors and co-editors, but only one has focused on masculinities—in the context of men's health (Gough and Robertson 2009). For a number of years I have been working with colleagues on a variety of topics concerning men and masculinities, ranging from male cosmetic use to accounts of depression, resulting in many journal articles, book chapters, and talks. But I have not yet had the opportunity to try to tie all this work together, and feel that to do so would explicate some implicit themes and issues which could advance the field—hence the reason for this book. So, I will attempt to articulate what I have learnt about masculinities over the years while being involved in different research projects.

For context, to help frame the book, it makes sense to say something about my background and approach. I am a social psychologist by training but engage with work from other social science disciplines (e.g. sociology) and interdisciplinary fields (including, notably, critical studies of men and masculinities), and have published in diverse places, such as health, sociology, and gender studies journals. I am currently co-editor of the APA journal *Psychology of Men & Masculinity*, with a brief to promote articles from outside Psychology and using a range of methods and theories. The book with Steve Robertson (Gough and Robertson 2009) is an edited volume which features contributions from media studies, nursing, sport science, and sociology, among others. Like many scholars in the field of men and masculinities, I have been influenced by the work of Connell (1995; Connell and Messerschmidt 2005) while also engaging with critiques of hegemonic masculinity and other concepts, mainly developed by sociologists, such as inclusive masculinity (Anderson 2009), pastiche masculinity (Atkinson 2010), and hybrid masculinity (Bridges and Pascoe 2012). Within social psychology, the seminal work of Wetherell and Edley (e.g. 1999) has had a marked impact on my research and thinking, encouraging close attention to the discourse practices of men and to locally pertinent norms of masculinity.

I am also a qualitative researcher and champion of qualitative research methods within Psychology and beyond. As co-founder and co-editor of the journal *Qualitative Research in Psychology*, I have endeavoured to promote quality, diversity, and innovation in qualitative methods. My own approach to research could be summed up as constructionist, psychosocial, and inductive: prioritising participant perspectives and locating these within relevant contexts, both proximal (i.e. research context and dynamics) and distal (e.g. wider gender norms and constraints). In recent years, I have moved beyond interview and focus group research to embrace other methods and data sources, in particular digital materials. This shift has been mainly prompted by my postgraduate students and early career colleagues engaged with social media, user-generated accounts (e.g. vlogs), and online interactions (e.g. support forums), and follows trends in the field towards more creative, multi-media, and 'naturalistic' research designs (e.g. Gough and Lyons 2016; Braun et al. 2017). In particular, we have found that many men, including hard-to-reach groups, are willing to provide accounts of their experiences and practices online, so many research examples cited in the book will derive from digital data.

In terms of research topics, I suppose I have been fascinated by studying men's sense-making in domains which have historically been dominated by women and thus considered feminised or feminising. So, the topics I have studied include men's accounts of diet, body image, and vulnerability. I have been intrigued to examine how men justify their engagement with 'the feminine' and the identity work that ensues: how do men who wear make-up/express emotion/ nurture others reproduce, rework, and reject masculinity norms? And what do these data signal about contemporary masculinities more generally—and current theories of masculinities?

This book interrogates conventional assumptions about masculinity and men's health and offers a coherent social-psychological position. It brings together in one place over a decade's work which showcases discursively inflected qualitative research using data sources where men's own accounts are prioritised, for example in-depth interviews and online discussion forums. It differs from previous men's health books which tend to be edited collections (e.g. Gough and Robertson 2009; Broom and Tovey 2009), while books on masculinity do not cover embodiment, emotions, or well-being in depth (e.g. Anderson 2009; Kahn 2009).

The book opens with a review of theory and research on contemporary masculinities; the second chapter looks at men's appearance concerns and activities; the third chapter covers male mental health, focusing on vulnerability and its management. The final chapter considers men's care for others (e.g. peers, partners), identifying ways in which men formulate support requests and responses, and how/why they champion certain groups (e.g. women; LGBT+ communities). The book concludes with an afterword, reflecting on current trends and key concepts, including intersectionality, inequalities, and embodiment.

Leeds, UK   Brendan Gough

References

Anderson, E. (2009). *Inclusive masculinity: The changing nature of masculinities.* New York: Routledge.

Atkinson, M. (2010). *Deconstructing men and masculinities.* Toronto: Oxford University Press.

Braun, V., Clarke, V., & Gray, D. (Eds.). (2017). *Collecting qualitative data: A practical guide to textual, media and virtual methods.* Cambridge: Cambridge University Press.

Bridges, T., & Pascoe, C. J. (2014). Hybrid masculinities: New directions in the sociology of men and masculinities. *Sociology Compass, 8*(3), 246–258.

Broom, A., & Tovey, P. (Eds.). (2009). *Men's health: Body, identity and social context.* Oxford: Wiley-Blackwell.

Connell, R. W. (1995). *Masculinities.* Cambridge: Polity Press.

Connell, R. W., & Messerschmidt, J. W. (2005). Hegemonic masculinity rethinking the concept. *Gender & Society, 19*(6), 829–859.

Gough, B., & Lyons, A. (2016). The future of qualitative research in psychology: Accentuating the positive. *IPBS: Integrative Psychological & Behavioral Science, 50*(2), 243–252.

Gough, B., & Robertson, S. (Eds.). (2009). *Men, masculinities and health: Critical perspectives.* Basingstoke: Palgrave.

Kahn, J. (2009). *An introduction to masculinities.* Oxford: Wiley Blackwell.

Wetherell, M., & Edley, N. (1999). Negotiating hegemonic masculinity: Imaginary positions and psycho-discursive practices. *Feminism & Psychology, 9*(3), 335–356.

Acknowledgements

Research is a collaborative effort and I would like to thank all colleagues and students I have worked with over the years on various projects concerning men and masculinities, including Steve Robertson, Esmee Hanna, Matthew Hall, Sarah Grogan, Sarah Seymour-Smith, Antonia Lyons, and Glen Jankowski—especially Steve and Esmee who kindly gave me valuable feedback on an earlier draft.

CONTENTS

CHAPTER 1

Theorising Masculinities

Abstract This chapter reviews influential theories of masculinity within Psychology and Critical Studies of Men and Masculinity. A social constructionist, psychosocial stance is advanced which emphasises how particular masculinities are constrained and enabled within particular contexts, intersected by other relevant identities such as social class, race, and sexual orientation. The importance of considering men as embodied, emotional, and caring is emphasised, that is, studying how men are engaging with traditionally feminised ideals and practices. As such, qualitative research focusing on local enactments of masculinities within specific communities is advocated, including online environments which may encourage more expansive expressions of (digital) masculinities. A focus on social change is articulated, situating (changing) men and masculinities at the forefront of gender equality and combating sexism and homophobia.

Keywords Masculinities • Theory • Social constructionist • Psychosocial • Intersectionality

In recent years 'masculinity' has been associated with various social phenomena ranging from male suicide to homophobia and (more positively) involved fathering and caring for others. Masculinity has attracted the attention of the public and scholars alike, provoking debates and crisis talk in the media as well as much theorising and research by social and human scientists. This chapter will critically consider some of the most influential theoretical work developing a framework which informs the other chapters in this book and which could be adopted (and adapted) by other researchers in the field. As a (social/critical) psychologist I will begin with psychological theories of men and masculinity (PMM) emanating from the USA before moving on to the interdisciplinary (though often sociological) field known as critical studies of men and masculinity (CMM). Although in my own work I have mainly been influenced by work within CMM I have more recently had the opportunity to engage with key concepts generated by colleagues working from a PMM tradition.

THE PSYCHOLOGY OF MEN AND MASCULINITY

Within Social and Personality Psychology the 'trait' approach to gender was dominant up until the 1980s, an approach which mapped biological sex directly onto gender identity; in other words, only men could be masculine and women feminine. This association between sex and gender began to be decoupled by Sandra Bem and colleagues—on the Bem Sex Role Inventory masculinity and femininity were formulated as independent constructs such that men could score on femininity and women on masculinity, with a high score on both dimensions producing an 'androgynous' sex role orientation (Bem 1974). However, trait theories and measures did not engage with how society constructed, (de)valued, and distributed gendered roles; there was no account of gendered power relationships and differentials. Subsequently, other psychologists influenced by feminism and men's liberation movements became more interested in the social construction of gender, and, specifically, the negative effects of masculinity norms/ ideologies on men (and others), initially conceptualised as gender role strain (GRS: Pleck 1981). In an early and influential piece, Brannon (1976) identified four traditional masculine norms:

- *No Sissy Stuff*: Men must avoid any behaviour or characteristic associated with women or femininity.
- *Be a Big Wheel*: Masculinity is measured by success, power, and receiving the admiration of others.
- *Be a Sturdy Oak*: Manliness is predicated on rationality, toughness, and self-reliance.
- *Give 'em Hell*: Men must balance the 'rationality' of the sturdy oak with daring and aggression, and must be willing to take risks in order to become the big wheel.

According to Pleck (1981), men are socialised to conform to dominant masculinity ideologies—with negative consequences, or gender role strain. When men successfully conform to the dominant masculinity norms this will have come at a cost to self and others (e.g. work immersion may cause stress and ill-health for the man and a compromised home life), while not living up to existing ideals may lead to feelings of failure and related self-esteem issues (Pleck 1981). This Gender Role Strain Paradigm (GRSP) pioneered by Pleck and colleagues has become very influential in the PMM in the USA (e.g. Wong et al. 2010). Trait measures of gender/masculinity have largely been rejected in favour of normative scales which measure the extent to which men endorse traditional masculinity ideals, such as the original Male Role Norm Scale (MRNS: Thompson and Pleck 1986). Two different scales have since been developed: one measuring conformity to norms, the Conformity to Masculine Norms Inventory (CMNI; Mahalik et al. 2003), and one assessing endorsement of norms, the Male Role Norms Inventory-Revised (MRNI-R; Levant et al. 2010). Research using the GRSP and associated measures has generally found that greater acceptance of and/or adherence to traditional masculinity ideologies (e.g. 'pursuit of status'; 'risk-taking'; 'self-reliance') is linked to a host of negative outcomes, ranging from sexism and homophobia (e.g. Parrott 2009) to health-averse practices (Hamilton and Mahalik 2009; Levant et al. 2011).

Influenced by the GRSP, other psychologists developed the concept of Gender Role Conflict (GRC: O'Neill 1981) to describe the unwelcome consequences of narrowly defined traditional masculinity ideals. To measure such outcomes, a Gender Role Conflict Scale (GRCS) has been designed (O'Neill et al. 1986) which identifies four main patterns in its factor analysis: Success/Power/Competition (SPC); Restrictive Emotionality (RE); Restrictive Affective Behaviour Between Men (RABBM) and Conflict Between Work and Family Relations (CBWFR). In a major review of empirical research using the GRCS, O'Neill (2008) indicates that 'GRC is significantly related to men's psychological and interpersonal problems' (358) while also being implicated in health-defeating practices such as excessive alcohol consumption.

In sum, US psychologists have developed an understanding of masculinity which is multifaceted, socially situated, and linked to a repertoire of negative consequences, including unhealthy practices. There is also a great concern with studying masculinity with respect to diverse communities, including marginalised groups such as Latino men, gay men, black men, disabled men, and men from disadvantaged backgrounds (e.g. Treadwell and Young 2012; Griffith et al. 2011)—this is reflected in the name change of Division 51 of the American Psychological Association (APA) from 'Psychology of Men and Masculinity' to 'Psychology of Men and Masculinities'. Much of the psychological research on masculinity has employed the normative measures mentioned above although, increasingly, psychologists focusing on men and masculinity are using qualitative methods and mixed method designs (e.g. Silverstein et al. 2002; Sloan et al. 2015). In addition, there is now more evidence that specific masculinity factors are associated with more positive outcomes, including health benefits for men (see Levant et al. 2011). This greater openness to methodological diversity, plurality masculinities, and the complexity of relationships between specific masculinity dimensions and health practices chimes with the work conducted outside US psychology.

Critical Studies of Men and Masculinity

Hegemonic Masculinity

Outside Psychology, masculinity theory has been particularly advanced by sociologists within the interdisciplinary field 'Critical Studies of Men and Masculinity' with a focus on societal and cultural constructions of masculinity and their impact on different groups of men (and women). Indeed, there has been some debate about the utility of the concept of masculinity/masculinities, with some arguing that it often homogenises men and encourages a fixed, reductionist outlook which draws attention away from what men actually do in practice (e.g. Hearn 2004, 1996). Nonetheless, the concept has endured and, arguably, now encompasses men's actions as well as social norms, most notably in relation to 'hegemonic masculinity' (Carrigan et al. 1985; Connell 1995; Connell and Messerschmidt 2005).

Hegemonic masculinity is not (only) about men and/or masculinity, but encompasses gender identities, relations, and conflicts—the gender order more widely. Early definitions emphasise this point: 'the currently most honoured way of being a man, it required all other men to position themselves in relation to it, and it ideologically legitimated the global subordination of women to men' (Connell and Messerschmidt 2005: 832). As such, a pluralistic and hierarchical perspective is presented where multiple masculinities (and feminities) exist and operate in relation to each other. Specifically, Connell highlighted the operation of power through masculinities, which are best understood as 'configurations of practice'; at a given moment in a given context some men will enact and be privileged by locally 'hegemonic' masculinities while women and other men will be marginalised or subordinated by these hegemonic practices. Opposition to and oppression of women and gay men (among others) are built into hegemonic masculinities. Disabled men may be marginalised through having limited access to material resources and valued masculinities. Similarly, gay men, oppressed by heterosexism and homophobia and judged to fall short of 'masculine' standards, are subordinated in both representational and material terms. For example, the discrimination, prejudice, and oppression faced by disadvantaged men have a deleterious impact on health and well-being (Griffith et al. 2011).

But individual men will experience a range of situations and relationships and in some contexts will take up (or will be assigned) more powerful positions while being placed in subordinated or marginalised positions in other contexts. For example, a manager may assume more power within an organisation compared to a security guard but this could be reversed in other circumstances (e.g. drinking or sporting scenarios). So, individuals may embody aspects of hegemonic masculinity in a particular setting, but may nonetheless be relatively disempowered through their positioning in other social contexts and structures. Thus material and cultural constraints often influence men's capacity to occupy hegemonic status; that is, engaging in particular configurations is not a matter of free choice. The embedding of gender within social structures is significant here as it is this that often facilitates or restricts access to a range of possible subject positions and access to material resources (Robertson et al. 2016).

The important concept of intersectionality is relevant here (Cole 2009), referring to the multiplicity of identities that an individual may embody pertaining to gender, social class, ethnicity, and so on—and the impact of different but related identity categories on individual experiences and opportunities. For example, as a white man certain privileges may well apply, but a white wheelchair user may experience a degree of emasculation relating to physical enactments of hegemonic masculinity (see Robertson 2007). Similarly, white working-class men who are unemployed may feel unable to occupy the traditionally treasured breadwinner role (Dolan 2007; Willot and Griffin 1997). Intersectionality cautions us against homogenising groups; not only is it simplistic to present men as a unified group, but also 'white working-class men' or 'black middle-class men'—intersectionality highlights complexity and nuance when considering questions of (masculine) identity, status, and well-being.

Returning to Connell, she also makes the point that many men may be 'complicit' with hegemonic masculinities—i.e. they may embody or concur with key features in particular contexts while not actively promoting or consciously subscribing to these hegemonic values. Connell (1995: 41) also uses the term 'patriarchal dividend' to suggest that all men gain in some way from the benefits that the structural embedding of hegemonic norms confers. So, Connell's theory of masculinity is relational as it concerns social comparisons, relative status, and competition. Central to Connell's approach is relations between men and women, since configurations of masculinities impact on women as well as men. For example, if masculinity has been defined around paid work outside the home (the traditional 'breadwinner' role), then women have been positioned, representationally and materially, within the household and as responsible for childcare and domestic labour.

Changing Masculinities?

To date, most work applying Connell's concepts—and indeed the psychological research on masculinity—has overwhelmingly focused on negative aspects/impacts of conventional masculinities. This preoccupation with the costs of masculinity has led some to alternative concepts which paint a more positive picture. For example, inclusive masculinity theory (Anderson 2014) contends that recent generations of (young) men have become less invested in traditional ('orthodox') masculine values and instead espouse a softer, more liberal, and open version of masculinity:

> *male youth today are better dressed digital hippies. They are young men who have grown up with less interest in religion or soldiering. They have gay friends, and value solving problems through talking instead of fighting. They readily express what men of my generation would have considered a highly feminized notion of masculinity, and they have greatly expanded upon the gendered and sexual behaviors that are not only permissible, but expected of their friends. ... They express emotional love for each other, kiss each other, and cuddle in bed together.* (Anderson 2014: 6;9)

Others highlight the potential of conventional masculine values to produce benefits, such as MacDonald's (2011) notion of 'salutogenic masculinity', which emphasises the health-promoting consequences of, say, men's participation in sport and physical activity. Psychologists working in the USA are also beginning to examine the relationships between specific masculinity factors and health outcomes (e.g. Levant et al. 2011). The concept of 'caring masculinity' (e.g. Elliott 2016) suggests an expansion of emotional expressiveness and care for others in men, for example in the realm of fathering, where there is often an effort to progress from the distant relationships that men have experienced with their own fathers. An interview study by Hanlon (2012: 203) in Ireland found that becoming involved in caring, for example for children, invariably led men to an enriched and expanded repertoire of masculinities:

> *Doing caring [...] appeared to support men to develop a 'softer' masculinity, to reform their lives and construct other-centred sensibilities, and to engage with fears surrounding vulnerability. It also enabled them to identify women's caring burdens and appreciate how difficult, complex, and underappreciated caring work can be.* (Cited in Elliott 2016)

Another strand of work on changing masculinities concerns men's engagement with feminism and social change. While there have been examples of men engaging with feminist movements throughout history, in recent years there has been greater interest and activity in different countries. For example, the European Union (EU) funded a programme of work on 'The Role of Men in Gender Equality' (Scambor et al. 2014) which addressed equality initiatives within the home, at work, and within interpersonal relationships. There are now various national initiatives focused on engaging (young) men in gender equality practices, such as the Great Men project (https://www.great-men.org/), which offers workshops in schools to 'improve the experience of boys and girls at school and challenge negative gender stereotypes which affect boys' behavior, mental health and academic performance, as well as the ways in which they interact with young women'. There are other initiatives focused on supporting gay, lesbian, and bisexual peers, such as the Stonewall 'Straight Allies' workplace guide (http://www.stonewall.org.uk/sites/default/files/straight_allies.pdf) and offshoots which focus on how (straight) men can advocate for equality. For example, 'Sport Allies' is a charity which uses proceeds from the Warwick Rowers naked calendar sales to promote inclusion within sport, with the rowers taking an inclusive approach to masculinity:

> *We are standing naked in front of the world as men who are prepared to be vulnerable, who embrace people of every gender and sexuality, and who are not afraid to show our affection for each other.* (http://www.sportallies.org/the-mission/)

Arguably, however, Connell's theory does allow sufficiently for positive relationships and outcomes associated with masculinity ideals and practices. As a social theory, change is admissible to the extent that society changes and presents new opportunities for men to (re)construct their masculinities (see Connell and Messerschmidt 2005): what counts as hegemonic in one time or setting can and does shift, such that the dominant formulation of masculinity in one community may foster connectedness and tolerance rather than competition and division. Such values may be enacted within men's groups, for example, whether therapeutic, work-based, or sport teams. Perhaps one change of note here concerns men's orientation to health: traditionally, concern for one's health has not featured centrally in definitions of masculinity; indeed, being unhealthy (e.g. excessive alcohol consumption; poor diet; risk-taking) could be regarded as a way of enacting hegemonic masculinity (Courtenay 2000). However, contemporary society, which has been described as 'healthist' (Crawford 2006), actively positions individuals as responsible for their health and so for men, being unhealthy is increasingly untenable; to pursue health-promoting practices now is to present oneself as rational, moral, and masculine (see Gough and Robertson 2009).

Connell's work underpins the structural and material bases to configurations of masculinity, that is, the resources and institutions which support particular versions of masculinity—and particular men/groups. This sociological focus presents a valuable perspective on power relations between men and between men and women, emphasising system-led inequalities—while perhaps underplaying the potential for challenging and transforming masculinities and gender relations, and for examining complexities and contradictions within local contexts. Discourse analytic research by Wetherell and Edley (1999), for example, highlights three main identity positions ('psycho-discursive practices') fashioned by men in their interview research, including 'heroic', 'ordinary', and 'rebellious' configurations. They note that the heroic position, denoting traditional 'macho' values, was least popular, which on the surface could be taken as progress; however, they also note that 'ordinary' and 'rebellious' positions, which create distance between self and heroic/macho values, may actually reproduce another version of traditional masculinity founded on autonomy and rationality. Hence, considering the construction of masculinities *in situ* highlights complexity, fluidity, and function—any one man can be regarded as both hegemonic and non-hegemonic at the same time, as both resistant and complicit.

It is also worth attending to wider discourses and their take-up by men from different social backgrounds. Considering men's health, for example, men are faced with (at least) two key discourses: one which encourages self-care, help-seeking, and restraint, and another which foregrounds pleasure, autonomy, and risk-taking—a control–release dilemma, or 'don't care/should care' couplet (see Robertson 2007). Exactly how such dilemmas play out for men inhabiting different circumstances, bodies, and biographies is a live research question: we cannot presume that these issues are negotiated in the same way by, say, white able-bodied middle-class professional men and mixed-race, working-class disabled men. In-depth qualitative research is required to explore how individual men and communities grapple with masculinities in relation to the local resources at their disposal (and relevant constraints thereof)—what are the key (or 'hegemonic') dimensions of masculinity relevant to specific groups of men in a changing world, and to what extent do they reinforce, rework, or reject conventional gender identities, practices, and relations?

Some theorists depart from Connell's theory to underline the plurality, flexibility, and fluidity of contemporary masculinities, as indicated by terms such as 'hybrid' (Bridges and Pascoe 2014), 'inclusive' (Anderson 2005), or 'pastiche' (Atkinson 2010) masculinity. In general, it is argued that boys and men are embracing skills, practices, and values once assigned (mainly) to women and femininity. For example, Anderson's work points to a softening of (heterosexual) masculinity whereby young men are comfortable in expressing affection for male peers and enjoy the company of women and gay friends. Although Anderson (2009) acknowledges that patriarchies still persist, he also deems it possible for men to relate to others *horizontally* (Anderson 2009; McCormack 2011), achieving status not through dominance, but through popularity. Whereas traditional masculinity operates through exclusion, specifically of the feminine or homosexual, inclusive masculinity, as the title suggests, accommodates and even integrates such qualities in order to develop more diverse strategies of achieving status (Anderson 2009; Bridges and Pascoe 2014). For example, McCormack's (2011) study involving 16- to 18-year-old males demonstrated how groups could establish and secure status by affecting qualities which garner admiration or even affection from others, for example emotional supportiveness.

Anderson's theory has been likened to post-feminism (O'Neill 2015) in its emphasis on personal choices and capacities rather than gendered power relations and constraints—an optimistic approach which skims over (ongoing) inequalities between men and women (and between men). In addition, how far inclusive masculinity is enacted outside a particular milieu (most of Anderson's research participants have been elite university 'jocks') remains to be seen. For example, the phenomenon has been criticised as restricted to certain cohorts of white Anglo-American middle-class university students (e.g. Ingram and Waller 2014). It can be suggested that men who enjoy privileged status and embody traditional markers of masculine success (e.g. in sport; work; wealth) can more easily engage in traditionally feminised practices without having their masculinity diminished (see Cleland 2013; O'Neill 2015). For example, de Visser et al. (2009) highlight how 'man points', or 'masculinity capital', can enable (young) men to resist masculinised practices (e.g. excessive alcohol consumption) and take up feminised pursuits (e.g. cooking) without censure. The concept is based upon Bourdieu's (1986) original theory of 'symbolic capital', which suggests that individuals accrue, lose, or trade the social 'credit' conferred by various aspects of experience, skill, understanding, and reputation, in furtherance of greater social status and authority (Bourdieu 1986). Similarly, masculine capital is a transactional system, within which individuals increase or decrease their masculinity 'score' by being awarded points for 'masculine' behaviours or penalised points for 'feminine' behaviours (de Visser and McDonnell 2013). For example, by abstaining from eating meat, vegetarian men risk losing masculine capital (Rothgerber 2012), but they may augment it by gaining points for athleticism (de Visser et al. 2009; de Visser and McDonnell 2013).

In my own work with colleagues looking at men's appearance practices we have noted a related tendency to account for feminised practices (e.g. wearing make-up) in masculinised terms (e.g. self-respect, success at work, female attraction; Hall et al. 2012a, b: see chapter 2). Another example: male patients, who previously may not have sought help in health-care settings in order to avoid any inference of weakness, may now reframe help-seeking as an act of bravery, defying one form of traditional masculinity (displaying weakness/seeking help) by invoking another (courage) in order to remain healthy and so be able to continue to support their families (Gough 2013). In other words, masculinity capital can be invoked to both facilitate and justify any activities that may be labelled unmanly or feminine. Some argue that, by taking on practices conventionally associated with marginalised others (women, gay men, and ethnic minorities), hegemonic masculinity is simply being repackaged by elite men in order to maintain power and privilege in a changing world: for example, middle-class white youth who appropriate 'gangsta rap' demeanours and symbols (see Bridges and Pascoe 2014; Demetriou 2001).

So, men today may find themselves in positions which their own fathers never or rarely had to inhabit, from more involved parenting to cooking and self-care. There now exists a range of new opportunities and challenges whereby men and boys might rethink their masculinity, perhaps making it easier in some instances to reject conventional norms (e.g. concerning sexism, homophobia, violence) and engaging in hitherto neglected and traditionally feminised practices, such as caring for others, expressing a repertoire of emotions, and paying more attention to appearance. Because we live in a world where both conventional and emerging masculinity ideals are in play, building a masculine identity will inevitably involve manoeuvring between different and sometimes conflicting dimensions, trying to strike a balance that works within particular contexts. Arguably, more privileged heterosexual men may experience more freedom to experiment with, say, appearance in ways which only recently were regarded as taboo. How individual men situated in different domains (with different levels of constraint) construct masculinities and manage appearance and well-being concerns is a live research area which has produced some telling insights but with more potential for new knowledge.

'DIGITAL MASCULINITIES'

In the chapters that follow, then, the focus is on how (heterosexual) men are engaging with and accounting for conventionally feminised practices in order to explore how contemporary masculinities are being constructed. I focus mainly on embodied and affective practices, reporting how men describe and explain a range of phenomena, including weight loss, depression, and infertility. Employing a broadly discursive approach, attention is paid to men's own words and perspectives—how and why they make gender (masculinity) relevant when talking to each other. The work of Wetherell and Edley (e.g. 1999, 2014), with its emphasis on social interaction, discourse dynamics, and the 'psycho-discursive' practices deployed by men, has influenced my approach here. The research discussed is often drawn from online spaces which some men use to tell their stories, seek help and support, and offer advice and care to their peers. Such online interactions provide rich, valuable 'data' because they proceed naturalistically—without any interference from researchers—and reference issues and emotions that many men may not feel comfortable sharing offline. As such, the collection and analysis of online data can be contrasted with more mainstream qualitative research, which tends to be interview-based and (overly) influenced by researcher agendas (see Potter and Hepburn 2005). In fact, there are now trends away from traditional qualitative methods towards more creative approaches, including online methods (see Braun et al. 2017), or 'netnography' (Kozinets 2002).

The focus on online spaces where men may enjoy opportunities to 'do' masculinity in more expansive ways is enabled under a comforting cloak of anonymity, for example enabling the expression of emotions normally withheld, or reserved for partners. This is not to imply that the internet automatically or naturally potentiates the performance of progressive masculinities. In fact, there is much evidence of online harassment, abuse, and hate speech perpetrated by men and male-dominated communities. Another criticism relates to the persistence of traditional masculinities (O'Neill 2015) as demonstrated, for example, in instances of everyday sexism (everydaysexism.com), the consumption of pornography by young men (Flood 2010), heavy drinking cultures, and associated violence and injury (Iwamoto et al. 2011). For example, there are social media sites associated with many British universities which encourage male students to 'confess' stories of sexual conquest, harassment, and objectification of women in drinking contexts. The sociologist and masculinity scholar Michael Kimmel (2013) has been studying the discourses promoted by white male supremacist groups online, arguing that masculinities are central to the prejudice and discrimination perpetuated in cartoons, jokes, and arguments. So, 'digital masculinities' may be destructive rather than creative, negative rather than positive, closed rather than open. However, in light of evidence that in certain online communities men display an engagement with a broad range of masculinities which may benefit their health and well-being (and that of significant others), a focus on the positive side of digital masculinities may offer insights into how men's identities can be expanded.

There is evidence that in a range of online contexts, including support groups, YouTube tutorials, and vlogs, many men are developing their digital masculinities in a climate of mutual support. For example, recent research by Anderson (Morris and Anderson 2015) highlights specific vloggers (online video bloggers) as exemplars of inclusive masculinity, performing affection, friendship, and acceptance of diversity. The extent to which men reinvent themselves online, however, is an open question; certainly, in the research I have been involved with we see both continuities and change in the ways men present themselves online. So, while some men may open up more online, display vulnerability, seek help, and offer support to peers, in doing so they may frame their accounts with traditional notions of masculinity in mind. The act of, say, expressing emotions online may transgress and reconstruct masculinity—but the ways in which such acts are framed, rationalised, and contextualised may well invoke more traditionally masculine signifiers, such as pragmatism, rationality, and action orientation. For example, emotion categories may be minimised, construed metaphorically, or justified in terms of health/well-being.

One of the aims of this book is to convey the complexities and contradictions pertaining to the construction and negotiation of masculinities (online), highlighting the opportunities and constraints bearing on men's identity practices. Although many examples of masculinities research highlighted in the book derive from online sources, other more traditional forms of qualitative data are also referenced, including interviews with overweight and obese men (Gough et al. 2016) and focus groups with young men discussing body image issues (Jankowski et al. submitted). Across all data sets cited, the key point is that men's own voices and meanings are prioritised, pertaining to embodiment, emotions, relationships, and masculine identities.

References

Anderson, E. (2005). Orthodox and inclusive masculinity: Competing masculinities among heterosexual men in a feminized terrain. *Sociological Perspectives, 48,* 337–355.

Anderson, E. (2009). *Inclusive masculinity: The changing nature of masculinities.* New York: Routledge.

Anderson, E. (2014). *21st century jocks: Sporting men and contemporary heterosexuality.* Basingstoke: Palgrave.

Atkinson, M. (2010). *Deconstructing men and masculinities.* Toronto: Oxford University Press.

Bem, S. L. (1974). The measurement of psychological androgyny. *Journal of Consulting and Clinical Psychology, 42,* 155–162.

Bourdieu, P. (1986). The forms of capital. In I. Szeman & T. Kaposy, (Eds.). (2011) *Cultural theory: An anthology* (pp. 81–93). Chichester: John Wiley & Sons, Ltd.

Brannon, D. (1976). The male sex role: Our culture's blueprint for manhood and what it's done for us lately. In D. Brannon (Ed.), *The forty-nine percent majority: The male sex role.* Reading: Addison-Wesley.

Braun, V., Clarke, V., & Gray, D. (Eds.). (2017). *Collecting qualitative data: A practical guide to textual, media and virtual methods.* Cambridge: Cambridge University Press.

Bridges, T., & Pascoe, C. J. (2014). Hybrid masculinities: New directions in the sociology of men and masculinities. *Sociology Compass, 8*(3), 246–258.

Carrigan, T., Connell, R. W., & Lee, J. (1985). Toward a new sociology of masculinity. *Theory and Society, 14,* 551–604.

Cleland, J. (2013). Book review: Inclusive masculinity: The changing nature of masculinities. *International Review for the Sociology of Sport, 48*(3), 380–383.

Cole, E. R. (2009). Intersectionality and research in psychology. *American Psychologist, 64,* 170–180.

Connell, R. W. (1995). *Masculinities.* Cambridge: Polity Press.

Connell, R. W., & Messerschmidt, J. W. (2005). Hegemonic masculinity rethinking the concept. *Gender & Society, 19*(6), 829–859.

Courtenay, W. H. (2000). Constructions of masculinity and their influence on men's well-being: A theory of gender and health. *Social Science & Medicine, 50,* 1385–1401.

Crawford, R. (2006). Health as a meaningful social practice. *Health, 10*(4), 401–420.

de Visser, R. O., & McDonnell, E. J. (2013). 'Man points': Masculine capital and young men's health. *Health Psychology, 32*(1), 5–14.

de Visser, R. O., Smith, J. A., & McDonnell, E. J. (2009). 'That's not masculine': Masculine capital and health-related behaviour. *Journal of Health Psychology, 14*(7), 1047–1058.

Demetriou, D. Z. (2001). Connell's concept of hegemonic masculinity: A critique. *Theory & Society, 30*(3), 337–361.

Dolan, A. (2007). 'Good luck to them if they can get it': Exploring working class men's understandings and experiences of income inequality and material standards. *Sociology of Health and Illness, 29*(5), 1–19.

Elliott, K. (2016). Caring masculinities: Theorising an emerging concept. *Men & Masculinities, 19*(3), 240–259.

Flood, M. (2010). Young men using porn. In K. Boyle (Ed.), *Everyday pornographies*. London: Routledge.

Gough, B. (2013). The psychology of men's health: Maximizing masculine capital. *Health Psychology, 32*(1), 1–4.

Gough, B., & Robertson, S. (Eds.). (2009). *Men, masculinities and health: Critical perspectives*. Basingstoke: Palgrave.

Gough, B., Seymour-Smith, S., & Matthews, C. R. (2016). Body dissatisfaction, appearance investment and wellbeing: How older obese men orient to 'aesthetic health'. *Psychology of Men & Masculinity, 17*(1), 84–91.

Griffith, D., Allen, J. O., & Gunter, K. (2011). Social and cultural factors influence African American men's medical help seeking. *Research on Social Work Practice, 21*, 337–347.

Hall, M., Gough, B., & Seymour-Smith, S. (2012a). 'I'm METRO, NOT gay', a discursive analysis of men's make-up use on YouTube. *Journal of Men's Studies, 20*(3), 209–226.

Hall, M., Gough, B., & Seymour-Smith, S. (2012b). On-line constructions of metrosexuality and masculinities: A membership categorisation analysis. *Gender and Language, 6*(2), 379–403.

Hamilton, C. J., & Mahalik, J. R. (2009). Minority stress, masculinity, and social norms predicting gay men's health risk behaviors. *Journal of Counseling Psychology, 56*, 132–141.

Hanlon, N. (2012). *Masculinities, care and equality: Identity and nurture in men's lives*. Basingstoke: Palgrave.

Hearn, J. (1996). Is masculinity dead?: A critique of the concept masculinity/masculinities. In M. Mac an Ghaill (Ed.), *Understanding masculinities* (pp. 202–217). Buckingham: Open University Press.

Hearn, J. (2004). From hegemonic masculinity to the hegemony of men. *Feminist Theory, 5*(1), 49–72.

Ingram, N., & Waller, R. (2014). Degrees of masculinity: Working and middle class undergraduate students' constructions of masculine identities. In S. Roberts (Ed.), *Debating modern masculinities*. London: Palgrave Macmillan.

Iwamoto, D. K., Cheng, A., Lee, C. S., Takamatsu, S., & Gordon, D. (2011). 'Man-ing' up and getting drunk: The role of masculine norms, alcohol intoxication and alcohol-related problems among college men. *Addictive Behavior, 36*(9), 906–911.

Jankowski, G., Gough, B., Fawkner, H., Diedrichs, P.C., & Halliwell, E. (submitted). It affects me, it affects me not: The impact of men's body dissatisfaction.

Kimmel, M. (2013). *Angry white men: American masculinity at the end of an era*. New York: Nation Books/Perseus.

Kozinets, R. V. (2002). The field behind the screen: Using the method of netnography to research market-oriented virtual communities. *Journal of Consumer Research, 39*(1), 61–72.

Levant, R. F., Rankin, T. J., Williams, C., Hasan, N. T., & Smalley, K. B. (2010). Evaluation of the factor structure and construct validity of the male role norms inventory-revised (MRNI-R). *Psychology of Men & Masculinity, 11*, 25–37.

Levant, R. F., Wimer, D. J., & Williams, C. M. (2011). An evaluation of the psychometric properties of the health behavior Inventory-20 (HBI-20) and its relationships to masculinity and attitudes towards seeking psychological help among college men. *Psychology of Men and Masculinity, 11*, 26–41.

MacDonald, J. (2011). Building on the strength of Australian males. *International Journal of Men's Health, 10*, 82–96.

Mahalik, J. R., Locke, B., Ludlow, L., Diemer, M., Scott, R. P. J., Gottfried, M., & Freitas, G. (2003). Development of the conformity to masculine norms inventory. *Psychology of Men and Masculinity, 4*, 3–25.

McCormack, M. (2011). Hierarchy without hegemony: Locating boys in an inclusive school setting. *Sociological Perspectives, 54*(1), 83–101.

Morris, M., & Anderson, E. (2015). 'Charlie is so cool like': Authenticity, popularity and inclusive masculinity on YouTube. *Sociology, 49*(6), 1200–1217.

O'Neil, J. M. (1981). Patterns of gender role conflict and strain: Sexism and fear of femininity in men's lives. *Personnel and Guidance Journal, 60*, 203–210.

O'Neil, J. M., Helm, B., Gable, R., David, L., & Wrightsman, L. (1986). Gender role conflict scale (GRCS): College men's fears of femininity. *Sex Roles, 14*, 335–350.

O'Neill, J. (2008). Summarizing 25 years of research on men's gender role conflict using the gender role conflict scale: New research paradigms and clinical implications. *The Counseling Psychologist, 36*, 358–445.

O'Neill, R. (2015). Whither critical masculinity studies? Notes on inclusive masculinity theory, Postfeminism, and sexual politics. *Men and Masculinities, 18*(1), 100–120.

Parrott, D. J. (2009). Aggression toward gay men as gender role enforcement: Effects of male role norms, sexual prejudice, and masculine gender role stress. *Journal of Personality, 77*, 1137–1166.

Pleck, J. (1981). *The myth of masculinity*. Cambridge, MA: MIT Press.

Potter, J., & Hepburn, A. (2005). Qualitative interviews in psychology: Problems and possibilities. *Qualitative Research in Psychology, 2*(4), 281–307.

Robertson, S. (2007). *Understanding men and health: Masculinities, identity and well-being*. Buckingham: Open University Press.

Robertson, S., Williams, B., & Oliffe, J. (2016). The case for retaining a focus on "masculinities" in Men's Health Research. *International Journal of Men's Health, 15*(1), 52–67.

Rothgerber, H. (2012). Real men don't eat (vegetable) quiche: Masculinity and the justification of meat consumption. *Psychology of Men & Masculinity, 14*(4), 363–377.

Scambor, E., Bergmann, N., Wojnicka, K., Belghiti-Mahut, S., Hearn, J., Holter, O. G., Gärtner, M., Hrženjak, M., Scambor, C., & White, A. (2014). Men and gender equality: European insights. *Men & Masculinities, 17*, 552–577.

Silverstein, L. B., Auerbach, C. F., & Levant, R. F. (2002). Contemporary fathers reconstructing masculinity: Clinical implications of gender role strain. *Professional Psychology, Research and Practice, 33*, 361–369.

Sloan, C. E., Gough, B., & Conner, M. T. (2015). How does masculinity impact on health? A quantitative study of masculinity and health behavior in a sample of UK men and women. *Psychology of Men & Masculinity, 16*, 206–217.

Thompson, E. H., & Pleck, J. H. (1986). The structure of male role norms. *American Behavioral Scientist, 29*, 531–543.

Treadwell, H. M., & Young, A. M. W. (2012). The right US men's health report: High time to adjust priorities and attack disparities. *American Journal of Public Health, 103*, 5–6.

Wetherell, M., & Edley, N. (1999). Negotiating hegemonic masculinity: Imaginary positions and psycho-discursive practices. *Feminism & Psychology, 9*(3), 335–356.

Wetherell, M., & Edley, N. (2014). A discursive psychological framework for analyzing men and masculinities. *Psychology of Men & Masculinities*, 355–365.

Willott, S., & Griffin, C. (1997). 'Wham, bam, am I a man?': Unemployed men talk about masculinities. *Feminism & Psychology, 7*(1), 107–128.

Wong, J., Steinfeldt, J., Hickman, S., & Speight, Q. (2010). Content analysis of the psychology of men & masculinity (2000–2008). *Psychology of Men & Masculinity, 11*, 170–182.

CHAPTER 2

Embodied Masculinities: Men's Body Projects

Abstract This chapter concerns men's discourse and practice around appearance, drawing on qualitative research studies featuring men's accounts of their body projects, including weight management and cosmetic use. This work is first contextualised with reference to relevant theoretical literature (e.g. sociology of the body; men and body image) and previous studies of male body dissatisfaction and 'metrosexual masculinities'. The data presented largely derive from online spaces where men talk to each other about practices such as diet, grooming, substance use, and make-up application, and highlight how men's accounts are simultaneously influenced by traditional and modern masculinity norms. While more men are engaging in conventionally feminised behaviours, it is clear that such behaviours are often reconstructed in 'masculine terms'. Implications for improving men's body image are discussed.

Keywords Appearance • Body image • Muscularity • Metrosexual • Body projects

Although most research to date on 'body image' has been conducted with women, it is increasingly recognised that men too worry about their bodies and engage in various practices in attempts to mitigate their concerns (e.g. Grogan 2008; Drummond 2011; Ricciardelli et al. 2006). While much of the research focusing on men has recruited younger men and has emphasised issues around muscularity (Pope et al. 2000), researchers are beginning to look at other groups of men (e.g. older men: Gough et al. 2016; men experiencing illness, e.g. prostate cancer: Drummond and Gough in press) and a wider range of issues, including hair, height, body shape, skin, and so on (e.g. Jankowski et al. submitted). This chapter reviews work on men and body image before presenting data on men's accounts relating to embodiment and appearance (mainly, muscularity, weight management, and cosmetic use). The place and meaning of masculinities within men's accounts of appearance practices will be discussed, and implications for addressing body image issues in men addressed.

MEN, MASCULINITIES, AND BODY IMAGE

Traditionally, men do not (much) care about their appearance; it is women who have been pressurised to focus on fashion, body shape and weight, hairstyle, skin, and so on and to invest in a range of products, services, and activities to maintain and enhance their appearance (see e.g. Bordo 1993). This is changing. The 1980s witnessed the emergence of male bodies as objects of desire across a range of media (magazine covers; billboards; television advertisements), when consumption began to be 'redefined as an activity that is suitable for men – rather than simply a passive and feminised activity' (Moore 1989: 179). Various explanations have been put forward to account for this shift, crediting fashion and image influences from the gay movement (Simpson 1994, 2002), equality pressures from feminist movements (Collier 1992), marketers seeking new avenues in late capitalist consumer societies (Featherstone 1991), and the advent of the style press confronting men on a daily basis with stylised images of other men's bodies (celebrity actors and models) linked to advertisements for men's products (Gill et al. 2005). Now there is ample evidence that men are investing in their appearance. Although there are historical and modern precedents where groups of men have experimented with appearance, such as the seventeenth-century Fop, eighteenth-century Macaroni, nineteenth-century Dandy, and various twentieth-century subcultures (teddy boys, mods, glam rockers, new romantics, etc.), these examples have been confined to particular communities and places. Now, we live in a society where image matters, where all individuals (men and women) are compelled to engage in various body projects in pursuit of desired images. The body is now a key resource for making and remaking identities in consumerist and individualistic cultures (Featherstone 1991; Giddens 1991; Shilling 1993). Individuals have become responsible for designing their bodies and, by extension, their identities. Since men have been traditionally marked as disembodied and rational (Seidler 1994), the increased visibility of and attention to male bodies may well provoke anxieties around body image (see Grogan 2008). On the other hand, masculinity has been inextricably tied to embodiment, typically in labour and sporting contexts (Connell 1995), and a renewed emphasis on the body may also present opportunities for embodied display and enhancement.

Watson (2000) has presented a useful model for thinking about men's embodiment. Based on interviews and observations at a well man's clinic, he identified four forms of embodiment referenced by male patients and health professionals. For example, while the men largely focused on 'pragmatic embodiment', that is how they could accomplish physical tasks, the clinic staff emphasised 'visceral embodiment', that is medical aspects such as blood pressure and heart rate. 'Normative embodiment', relating to bodily appearance, and 'experiential embodiment', where the body engenders feelings, were not much invoked by staff or patients. Another interview-based study by Gill et al. (2005) found that men emphasised autonomy and control, presenting themselves as 'the individual managers of their own bodies' (2005: 55). These and other studies reinforce the significance of masculinity norms which privilege bodily functionality and achievement over feminised emotions (e.g. Seidler 1994). However, other research suggests a more complex picture. For example, in Robertson's (2006) interview study, the male interviewees referenced all four of Watson's embodiment repertoires (pragmatic; experiential; visceral; and normative) when talking about their health and lifestyles. Another study by Robertson and colleagues (Robertson et al. 2010), this time with men on a cardiac rehabilitation programme, found that men deployed an experiential account where feelings concerning the body are disclosed—an 'embodied emotionality'. For example, improving fitness via the exercise component of the cardiac rehabilitation programme was seen to confer benefits experientially (feeling good), pragmatically (task completion), normatively (looking good), and viscerally (e.g. lower cholesterol readings).

In terms of body image, the ubiquitous body ideal for men across many Western societies is lean and muscular (Grogan 2008). Combined with a societal demonisation of overweight and obese bodies (Monaghan 2008), many boys and men may feel pressure to work on their bodies, for example through physical activity, diet, and substance use. But the current ideal extends beyond body fat and muscularity and specifies norms around hair, body hair, skin tone, height, penis size, and so on (Jankowski et al. 2014). There is growing evidence that the contemporary preoccupation with appearance is impacting boys and men. Questionnaire studies typically find that at least 35% of male respondents report dissatisfaction in relation to body fat, muscularity, height, and so on (e.g., Liossi 2003; Mellor et al. 2010). Such dissatisfaction has been noted in younger populations, including boys as young as eight years old (Grogan 2008). More men report dissatisfaction than have ever before (Gray and Ginsberg 2007), which has been increasingly linked to a range of psychological problems, from depression to eating disorders (Olivardia et al. 2004; Bordo 1999; Pope et al. 2000). Pope and colleagues (2000), for instance, found that men who frequented the gym, and reported muscle dissatisfaction, often followed strict, limited eating regimes that interfered with their work and social lives. A further well-documented impact of men's body dissatisfaction is the non-medical use of anabolic-androgenic steroids (Kanayama et al. 2006). A large meta-analysis of studies assessing steroid prevalence found that the lifetime prevalence of steroid use among men and boys was 7% (Sagoe et al. 2014) and other research has suggested their prevalence is increasing (Advisory Council on the Misuse of Drugs 2010; Hall et al. 2015). Thought to cause fat-free mass gain, little attention is heeded to steroids' numerous health risks by the men who resort to their use. Such health problems include elevated risk of cardiovascular disease, significant psychological disturbances, and cognitive impairment (Advisory Council on the Misuse of Drugs 2010; Pope et al. 2000).

Older men are not immune; for example, increasing numbers of middle-aged and older men are participating in fitness programmes and events, including marathons, 'ironman' competitions, and bodybuilding (e.g. Phoenix and Sparkes 2009). There is also some evidence that corporations are setting appearance-based expectations for male executives (Miller 2005). Men may also experience body dissatisfaction when dealing with a medical condition and/or its treatment. For example, treatment for prostate cancer through surgery may leave a man with erectile dysfunction, while Androgen Deprivation Therapy (ADT), which is said to 'chemically castrate' men by reducing the amount of testosterone that is produced by the male body; in both cases, men experience body image issues linked with masculinity (Filiault et al. 2008). Being overweight or diagnosed as obese may also produce body dissatisfaction in men (see Gough et al. 2016), with specific issues such as gynaecomstia ('man boobs') also causing distress in men (Singleton et al. 2009).

The significance of male body image is underlined by the now staggering range of products and services marketed to men, including body hair removal (e.g. waxing, electrolysis, tweezing, threading), body tanning and artwork, skincare products (facial and body moisturisers, anti-aging and fatigue creams and gels), cosmetics ('manscara', 'guyliner', face powder, blusher, lip gloss, illuminator), self and specialist teeth-whitening, cosmetic surgery procedures including major (rhinoplasty, rhytidectomy), minor (mole, tattoo, and cyst excision), self-administrable (Botox, chicken pills, Hydrogel), and lunchtime procedures (laser liposuction) (see Aitkenhead 2005). It is clear that men today have a range of options for addressing perceived bodily shortcomings, from everyday items available on the high street to more radical 'solutions' such as cosmetic surgery and use of diverse substances. But, how do men themselves account for their appearance-related practices, and how is masculinity constructed and negotiated with reference to body image? Specifically, how do men manage to navigate between conventional masculine norms which emphasise bodily function and strength, and mind over body—and current ideals which promote appearance investment and particular bodily configurations (lean, muscular, smooth, etc.)? Below, I explore these questions in relation to stereotypical (e.g. physical activity) and modern (e.g. cosmetic use) body projects for men.

It is worth noting that boys and men are often reluctant to talk about their bodies or sources of body dissatisfaction. For example, Taylor (2011) noted in her ethnographic research that her US male participants could not be seen to be emotionally affected by others' appearance teasing whereas Ricciardelli et al. (2006) noted a similar reluctance in their Australian high school male participants, which boys and men themselves attribute to masculinity norms, anxieties about appearing unmasculine, weak, and 'uncool' (Adams et al. 2005), or vain (Gill et al. 2005). Admitting body dissatisfaction is difficult for men, it seems, not because they do not have it, but rather because it contravenes standards of hegemonic masculinity. For this reason we have tended to research men's accounts of body practices in online environments, where of course they can (and do) tell their stories anonymously.

Muscularity and Weight Management Projects

Research on embodiment and self-image is emerging which reinforces this picture of boys finding it difficult to deal with bodily imperfections in the context of peer surveillance, idealized media images, and sports and physical education cultures which prioritise hard, masculinised bodies and practices (e.g. Kehler and Atkinson 2010). As noted above, many boys and (young) men are oriented to pursue a lean, muscular ideal—a traditionally masculine way of doing body work. Psychologists have devised a scale called the Drive for Muscularity (DFM: McCreary and Sasse 2000), which has been used to estimate prevalence of this issue (high) and link DFM to a range of problems, such as low self-esteem and anxiety (Edwards et al. 2014). DFM is also unsurprisingly linked to weight training, supplement intake, and nutrition regimes designed to add mass, practices which can become extreme and health-threatening (Edwards et al. 2014).

Our own work (Hall et al. 2015) has studied how (young) men account for their ingestion of appearance-enhancing substances such as synthol and ephedrine. For example, ephedrine is marketed as a weight loss supplement, often in conjunction with caffeine and aspirin (the ECA stack), and is popular with bodybuilders and other gym users (mostly male) who want to achieve a lean and muscular look (see Ricciardelli 2012). In our study we found that contributors to an online forum on ephedrine use tended to emphasise benefits and downplay risk, side effects, or longer-term health implications:

R8:   *i take eph regularly, awesome, and i have noticed the fat loss while on it! i took some this morning and will take another dose about 12 or 1 i dont get much sides, a little jittery but i enjoy it, also feel the adrenaline pumping from about 7am-10am lol.*

Here, a range of physical benefits are emphasised, with side effects minimised ('a little jittery') and no mention of health concerns. In fact, various health problems have been associated with ephedrine, including anxiety, restlessness, and insomnia, with sustained use possibly leading to myocardial infarction and stroke (Calfee and Fadale 2006). Additionally, we know that such substances can produce addiction issues with young male steroid users (Smith et al. 2016), as well as 'muscle dysmorphia', a preoccupation with minimising body fat and maximising muscularity (Murray et al. 2010).

In a parallel study of synthol use the findings were similar (Hall et al. 2015). Synthol is an oil-based substance which can be injected directly into specific muscles for augmentation purposes (Childs 2007). In our study the endurance of pain associated with injecting was normalised; in response to a question on this subject, other forum contributors unanimously minimised the discomfort involved and accentuated the positive effects:

Yes, that is normal. The pain will be less and less each day until after the first week you will not feel it anymore. Synthol is great stuff. You will be pleased.

It is difficult to determine the prevalence of such substance use for appearance purposes, but from our work and other research in this area we know that (young) men are prioritising a lean and muscular appearance often with scant regard for the potential impact on health and well-being.

For those men and boys who are overweight or classified as obese, losing weight can become important for their body confidence and masculine identity as much as for health benefits. In our interview study with men who were participating in a local weight management programme (Gough et al. 2016), our interviewees expressed a range of negative emotions connected to their oversized bodies, for example:

I'm very conscious of my weight, hate it, I'm not one of these happy fat blokes I really am not ... absolutely not. (John, age 63)

The self-disgust goes with it and that winds things down. (Jim, age 63)

In the men's accounts of their subsequent weight loss journeys, they highlighted appearance- related and psychological benefits over and above health ones:

losing the weight has been great I've noticed my belt goes up a couple of notches and clothes are fitting better that's brilliant. (Sam, 30)

I used to suffer with er anxiety and I haven't suffered with that since I lost weight. (Phil, 34)

The men expressed pride and satisfaction with their slimmer physiques, focusing on their new, improved appearance and better fitting clothes. In addition, achieving personal weight loss targets seems to bring about a transformation in body satisfaction and subjective well-being. These weight loss success stories echo those found in women's magazines and suggest that (these) men are comfortable within such feminised narratives.

In another study we found that men were quite happy to talk to other men online about their weight loss endeavours and their desired appearance (Bennett and Gough 2013). This appearance orientation can be linked to Crawshaw's (2007) notion of 'aesthetic health' whereby men are increasingly called upon as bodily subjects obliged to maintain disciplined, healthy, and attractive bodies. Many men on this online weight loss forum also expressed particular interest in getting rid of their '*bellies*', '*man boobs*', and '*saggy bits*'—a concern with stemming 'leaky' embodiment. We also found that the same men displayed an interest in maintaining or developing a more masculine look, in achieving their aspirations via masculinised activities, and in reaping the heteronormative benefits for their efforts. For example, some forum members construed their body projects in very technical terms:

> *I can see some changes in body shape, my delts are a separate entity again (shoulder balls), if I 'flex' I have noticeable biceps, my legs have some definition. The belly is cutting in and coming up. The visceral (hard belly fat, known to docs as heart attack fat) fat is noticeably decreased. The massive difference though is in my face. Starting to get a proper defined jaw line again.* (Richy 6)

Such accounts echo those from research on bodybuilding, where attention is also focused on acquiring an aesthetically pleasing body judged on muscular mass, symmetry, and definition (Roundtree 2005), a body from which individual bodybuilders can experience much satisfaction (Monaghan 2008). In the pursuit of manly bodies, the potentially feminising orientation to appearance is recuperated as a legitimate masculine concern. When communicating about food preparation a similar masculinising effort was in evidence, with the kitchen reimagined as a site for moulding muscular bodies:

> *I think the saying 'a sixpack is made in the kitchen and not in the gym' is 100% true.* (Jamie 15)

> *Be a beast in the gym and a beast in the kitchen, that's where good bodies are made.* (Richy 6)

Here, muscularity is first connected to the kitchen, which is then likened to the gym as a legitimate space for masculine endeavour ('be a beast') and the production of fit male bodies. This construction of cooking in a masculine way for weight-training purposes has been found in the wider media as a way to further reinforce hegemonic masculinity, for example through the use of military and evolutionary metaphors and the rise of celebrity male chefs (see Gough 2007). This study examined the discussions on an online forum linked to Men's Health magazine—a publication which idealises muscularity and provokes appearance concerns (e.g. Stibbe 2004; Labre 2005). It is therefore a very distinctive context where talk of muscularity and hard bodies is to be expected.

Yet, men's appearance anxieties and activities extend beyond pursuing a leaner and/or more muscular look. These days, men and boys are expected to attend to their skincare, hairstyle, body hair, and apparel, among other things. Men who are unhappy with their height, nose, ears, penis size, breasts, and so on may avail of various services and interventions, including cosmetic surgery. Men are increasingly targeted with more grooming products and services, including cosmetic ranges and 'manscaping' (body hair removal, e.g. through waxing). In our research on 'metrosexual masculinities', we have been interested to understand how (straight) men constructed their practices—and their masculine identities.

METROSEXUAL MASCULINITY: COSMETIC USE; MANSCAPING

Young, 'metrosexual' men most obviously care about their appearance. A metrosexual has been defined as

> *a young man with money to spend, living in or within easy reach of a metropolis – because that's where all the best shops, clubs, gyms and hairdressers are.* (Simpson 2002: 2)

Coad (2008) argues that the modern marketing of male sports stars and celebrities has given permission for men to care about their appearance; others argue that a shift in the labour market where self-presentation is important has generated new image-related expectations for men (e.g. Miller 2009). Whether or not male grooming represents a departure from—or merely a reworking of—traditional masculinity is an open question, one which we have investigated by analysing the accounts of self-identified metrosexual men. One of our studies focused on straight men who wear make-up (Hall et al. 2012a); specifically, their online posts relating to cosmetic practices. Briefly, our study considered how men responded to a YouTube tutorial delivered by a young man which was designed to provide advice and tips for other men. Immediately apparent from this video was the last section, where the presenter signed off with the words: 'BTW, I'm METRO not gay!' Obviously, doing something traditionally associated with women and femininity may create issues for masculine identity, and this is something we encountered with the online responses to the tutorial. For example, using make-up to create a 'masculine' effect was emphasised:

> *I think that maybe a bit more contouring such as bringing out the tops of your cheek bones the middle of your nose and your chin and forehead would make it a more masculine look. and darkening under the cheekbones and on the sides of the nose and up to the inside of the eyebrow would make you look more chiseled.* ☺

In general, although we found that the men talked (online) in detail about their routines and favourite products, they tended to stress practical benefits over beautification:

> *it's nice to see another guy like me who wears makeup. I wear mine because I have a mild form of rosacea.*
> *many straight men in Sydney Australia wears make up because we got harsh sun and windy winter down here. Even some NRL players I know wear makeup when they go out.*

Cosmetic use is here warranted by health rather than appearance concerns (rosacea—a skin condition), and with reference to the effects of a harsh climate on facial appearance. The first example presents a personal story while the second implicates many men—straight men, including those men who might be deemed privileged or stereotypically masculine: (Australian rules) football players. So, wearing make-up is ok for men if it is to cover up a skin complaint or to combat the impact of environmental conditions.

In addition, cosmetic use was also linked to heterosexual appeal and success, as evidenced in the next extract featuring a post regarding the YouTube make-up tutorial and a response from the tutorial creator:

> Post
> *hey bro good shit im right there wit ya … everymorning …*
> *my girlfriend loves having a guy who can look flawles :)*

Response (VC – Video Creator)
Niceeee! aha
Girls love it_ actually
x]

Invoking the 'girlfriend' and 'girls' in general situates make-up use as a legitimate practice for straight men because it can lead to admiration and attention from women, thus confirming male users as masculine, that is not effeminate or gay. As with our other studies on 'metrosexuality' (Hall et al. 2011, 2012b), our findings suggest that conventional masculinities are not in decline, but are merely being reworked and repackaged in a more image-conscious, consumer-oriented society. In particular, the emphasis on not appearing gay highlights the continued influence of homophobia with ostensible gender rebels, thus questioning claims regarding the declining significance of homophobia (McCormack 2012) and the advent of inclusive masculinities (Anderson 2005).

Another metrosexual activity traditionally associated with women is body hair removal, now colloquially known as 'manscaping' (see Immergut 2010). Images of male bodies in popular culture invariably depict smooth chests, with more men now attending salons for waxing purposes (Hall 2015). A recent trend here concerns the removal of hair around the genitals—a procedure which supposedly makes the penis appear longer. Indeed, a recent advertising campaign by Gillette promotes their razors for this very purpose: 'When there's no underbush the tree looks taller.' However, men who engage in this activity risk appearing unduly concerned about their penis size as well as appearing unduly interested in feminised body hair removal. In a recent study, Hall (2015) studied how men accounted for their groin shaving via online posts in response to the Gillette YouTube video 'how to shave down there'. The analysis highlighted the persistence of masculinity concerns within the men's accounts. For example, groin shaving was presented in terms of hygiene and aesthetics:

Most of us aren't trying to fool anyone. It's just getting it cleaner and free of unwanted hair. (Ontherodney)

Here genital hair removal is construed as normative ('most of us') and pragmatic—nothing to do with penis enlargement or feminised vanity (see

Gill et al. 2005). Alternatively, the practice was linked to heterosexuality and pleasure:

> *I really didn't want to do that but my girl said I had to or else I don't get any:(*
> (Sammyboy)

In this extract, genital hair removal is attributed to female exhortation, not a free choice but one which nonetheless pays dividends. A similar account linked the practice to gender equality:

> *Why should women be expected to keep it clean down there but not guys? Its respect. I don't like hair, and I'm sure women don't either. They appreciate a clean shaven man and I'm happy to give it them. Welcome to the 21st century.*
> (Silversimon)

Here, genital hairlessness is presented as a contemporary norm which includes men and women; again, women are positioned as favouring clean shaven men. Collectively, these repertoires work to masculinise a potentially transgressive practice by disavowing a penis enlargement rationale and foregrounding a commonplace practical and heterosexual-ised activity.

IMPLICATIONS

The research to date suggests that boys and men are invested in their appearance, with many reporting body dissatisfaction and some willing to talk about body image issues in environments perceived to be safe and supportive (e.g. online discussion forums). However, there is still much more research to be done. For example, we know little about men's every-day body anxieties beyond (younger) men's preoccupation with muscular-ity and (older) men's focus on weight management. Moreover, there is insufficient attention to body image issues in diverse male constituencies, including Black and Minority Ethnic men, disabled men, and working-class men. It is important to gain insights into the appearance concerns and practices of different communities so that relevant interventions can be designed where significant issues are identified. To date, most body image interventions have focused on women (e.g. Stice et al. 2008), with a few attending to gay men (e.g. Brown and Keel 2015). Any intervention applied to (straight) men will clearly have to attend to masculinity factors, both in terms of facilitating disclosure about appearance-related issues in the first instance and then engaging men in activities and discussions to challenge prevailing (gendered) body image ideals.

One of our recent projects attempted to facilitate disclosure of bodily anxieties and to promote critical awareness of prevailing appearance ideals among male university students (Jankowski et al. submitted). Here, we used a version of the Body Project M programme which had been used before with women/gay men (e.g. Brown and Keel 2015). The intervention comprised various components within a group discussion setting, such as icebreakers, identifying aspects of the current male beauty ideal, role plays, and asking critical questions about appearance norms. Between the two group sessions, participants were assigned homework tasks, including a challenge to change a current appearance behaviour and writing a letter to the younger self or a male relative about body image issues. During the group discussions, it was evident that the young men were reluctant to reveal any personal information about their body-related concerns, with most claiming that they were not affected by contemporary ideals and pressures. For example, Lee said at the start of his session:

I honestly can't think of [any appearance pressure] that annoys me. I was going to think of trying to say something but I can't even.

Others echoed this view:

Dustin: *To be honest it seems that none of us really care too much about our appearances.*
Robert: *Yeah*
Dustin: *It's like, what there isn't much that's stops us and that I'd say*

However, as rapport was developed within the focus groups, and the participants completed the intervention tasks, the discussion progressed to more personal revelations applied to a range of issues, including hair, weight, height, and skin. For example, some participants focused on hair-related issues:

I've actually not cut my hair for like 3 months or something because I'm just trying to get it to grow over the receding hairline … it does get to me … it's just the fact that you're losing your hair or going to lose your hair is just a demeaning thing. (Greg)

Researcher: *What if your (hair) straighteners broke?*
Robin: *I would cry ... I would order a new pair and not go out until they arrive. ... Mine have actually broken and I didn't go out until my new ones came first class post. (laughs)*

Here the young men highlight the emotional impact of hair problems ('demeaning'; 'I would cry') and reveal strategies for coping with these, both in the longer term (covering a receding hairline) and short-term (staying indoors awaiting new hair straighteners).

It would be interesting to follow up this sample to check for longer-term impact. More generally, to help promote greater engagement from boys and men it seems important to involve them in intervention design and content, that is participatory action research to identify key issues and possible ways forward from the 'inside'. A key component of such interventions might be to cultivate a critical awareness of corporate, media, and consumerist agendas in the perpetuation of gendered body ideals so that individuals do not blame themselves or each other for perceived shortcomings.

Other interventions directed at men have focused on one particular issue, for example weight management. As men tend not to access traditional corporate weight management groups and services, with 'dieting' perceived as feminised and women-centred (Bye et al. 2005), some recent initiatives have developed to encourage more men to adopt healthier lifestyles. For example, a series of men's health 'manuals' have been produced in the UK, sponsored by the Men's Health Forum, and styled in the format of a well-known car maintenance manual (e.g. Banks 2005). I analysed one such manual which targeted overweight and obese men and promoted healthy eating and exercise activities (Gough 2009). As with the previous studies of men's health promotion in UK newspapers citedsabove, I noted that, somewhat ironically, (overweight) male bodies were presented as machine-like, requiring regular maintenance (as a car would), that men were presented as disembodied thinkers who could use mental strength and logic to lose weight, and that their masculinity-related practices (eating red meat, drinking beer, etc.) should remain intact. Thus, men's health promotion becomes caught in a tension between providing dedicated advice and reinforcing aspects of masculinity associated with unhealthy lifestyles and poor health outcomes. The possible negative impact of reinforcing particular aspects of masculinity on public health more broadly has been highlighted elsewhere (Smith and Robertson 2008).

Beyond health promotion advice in print media, some obesity reduction initiatives have attempted to recruit men into programmes using more nuanced understandings of masculinity within these processes, such as drawing on the popularity and power of sport for many men (Gray et al. 2009). A recent health promotion intervention designed specifically for men, Football Fans in Training (FFIT), has proved successful with overweight men in Scotland (Hunt et al. 2014). This programme was supported by professional football clubs that offered their stadiums as sites for group-based work with overweight men; another strand of the programme entailed pedometer-based walking and physical activity sessions on the soccer field facilitated by club coaches. Qualitative interviews with the men post weight loss highlighted an appreciation of the pedometers as a tool for self-monitoring, a valuing of enhanced fitness within a male-friendly soccer space, and the associated masculine capital accrued (Hunt et al. 2014).

Beyond weight management, there is scope for the evaluation of existing initiatives and the creation of new ones focusing on other issues. For example, one established campaign in the UK revolves around men and eating disorders: mengeteatingdisorderstoo.co.uk. This charity features testimonies by men and provides peer support online, anonymously—the impact of these services has yet to be evaluated. It is not difficult to imagine similar initiatives for men experiencing other body image issues, for example relating to skin conditions, hair loss, height, and so on—and if there are initiatives out there already then they could be studied and evaluated to determine the benefits. It is also worth noting the increasing number of websites offering advice to men about make-up use (e.g. thebeautyboy.co.uk); again, these could be assessed for their utility. We also need interventions to help reduce the use of steroids and other appearance-modifying substances like ephedrine and synthol by (young) men in gym environments.

In sum, care needs to be taken in order to elicit stories from men about their bodies; men need to feel comfortable in order to self-disclose and to feel that they will not be criticised or considered unmasculine. As we have seen, online environments may be perceived as safe spaces where men can admit to a range of body image issues and receive peer support and advice. With face-to-face interventions, including participants as co-researchers to help design and test ideas can help make the intervention more relevant—

and more effective. Of course, programmes need to be tailored to particular groups; for example, with younger people drawing materials from social media for discussion purposes may work well. Knowledge of and sensitivity to the specific features and needs of communities is imperative, not least locally pertinent masculinities—what works for some groups of men may not work in others. For example, initiatives centred around sport will be effective in some constituencies while other men may prefer a focus on popular culture.

REFERENCES

Adams, G., Turner, H., & Bucks, R. (2005). The experience of body dissatisfaction in men. *Body Image, 2*(3), 271–283.

Advisory Council on the Misuse of Drugs. (2010). *Consideration of the anabolic steroids*. UK Government. Retrieved from https://www.gov.uk/government/publications/advisory-council-on-the-misuse-of-drugs-consideration-of-the-anabolic-steroids—2

Aitkenhead, D. (2005, September 14). Most British woman now expect to have cosmetic surgery in their lifetime: How did the ultimate feminist taboo become just another lifestyle choice? *The Guardian*, p. 13.

Anderson, E. (2005). Orthodox and inclusive masculinity: Competing masculinities among heterosexual men in a feminized terrain. *Sociological Perspectives, 48*, 337–355.

Banks, I. (2005). *The HGV man manual*. Somerset: Haynes Publishing.

Bennett, E., & Gough, B. (2013). In pursuit of leanness: Constructing bodies and masculinities online within a men's weight management forum. *Health, 17*(3), 284–299.

Bordo, S. (1993). *Unbearable weight: Feminism, western culture and the body*. Berkeley: University of California Press.

Bordo, S. (1999). *The male body: A new look at men in public and in private* (1st paperback ed.). New York: Farrar, Straus & Giroux Inc.

Brown, T. A., & Keel, P. K. (2015). A randomized controlled trial of a peer co-led dissonance-based eating disorder prevention program for gay men. *Behaviour Research and Therapy, 74*, 1–10.

Bye, C., Avery, A., & Lavin, J. (2005). Tackling obesity in men - preliminary evaluation of men only groups within a commercial slimming organization. *Journal of Human Nutrition and Dietetics, 18*, 391–394.

Calfee, R., & Fadale, F. (2006). Popular ergogenic drugs and supplements in young athletes. *Pediatrics, 117*, 577–589.

Childs, D. (2007). Like implants for the arms: Synthol lures bodybuilders. *ABC News*. Available at: http://abcnews.go.com/Health/Fitness/story?id=3179969

Coad, D. (2008). *The metrosexual: Gender, sexuality, and sport.* New York: State University of New York Press.

Collier, R. (1992). The new man: fact or fad? *Achilles Heel.* Retrieved June 6, 2009, from http://www.achillesheel.freeuk.com/article14_9.html

Connell, R. W. (1995). *Masculinities.* Cambridge: Polity Press.

Crawshaw, P. (2007). Governing the healthy male citizen: Men, masculinity, and popular health in Men's Health magazine. *Social Science & Medicine, 65,* 1606–1618.

Drummond, M. J. (2011). Reflections on the archetypal heterosexual male body. *Australian Feminist Studies, 26*(67), 103–117.

Drummond, M., & Gough, B. (in press). Men, body image and cancer. In M. Fingeret & I. Teo (Eds.), *Principles and practices of body image care for cancer patients.*

Edwards, C., Tod, D., & Molnar, G. (2014). A systematic review of the drive for muscularity research area. *International Review of Sport and Exercise Psychology, 7,* 18–41.

Featherstone, M. (1991). The body in consumer culture. In M. Featherstone, M. Hepworth, & B. S. Turner (Eds.), *The body: Social process and cultural theory* (pp. 170–196). London: Sage.

Filiault, S. M., Drummond, M. J., & Smith, J. (2008). Gay men and prostate cancer: Voicing the concerns of a hidden population. *Journal of Men's Health, 5*(4), 327–332.

Giddens, A. (1991). *Modernity and self-identity: Self and society in the late modern age.* Cambridge: Polity Press.

Gill, R., Henwood, K., & McLean, C. (2005). Body projects and the regulation of normative masculinity. *Body and Society, 11*(1), 39–62.

Gough, B. (2007). 'Real men don't diet': An analysis of contemporary newspaper representations of men, food and health. *Social Science & Medicine, 64*(2), 326–337.

Gough, B. (2009). Promoting `masculinity` over health: A critical analysis of Men's health promotion with particular reference to an obesity reduction `manual'. In B. Gough & S. Robertson (Eds.), *Men, masculinities and health: Critical perspectives.* Basingstoke: Palgrave.

Gough, B., Seymour-Smith, S., & Matthews, C. R. (2016). Body dissatisfaction, appearance investment and wellbeing: How older obese men orient to 'aesthetic health'. *Psychology of Men & Masculinity, 17*(1), 84–91.

Gray, J. J., & Ginsberg, R. L. (2007). Muscle dissatisfaction: An overview of psychological and cultural research and theory. In J. K. Thompson & G. Cafri (Eds.), *The muscular ideal: Psychological, social, and medical perspectives* (pp. 15–39). Washington, DC: American Psychological Association.

Gray, C., Anderson, A., Dalziel, A., Hunt, K., Leishman, J., & Wyke, S. (2009). Addressing male obesity: An evaluation of a group-based weight management intervention for Scottish men. *Journal of Men's Health and Gender, 6*, 70–81.

Grogan, S. (2008). *Body image: Understanding body dissatisfaction in men, women, and children.* London: Routledge.

Hall, M. (2015). 'When there's no underbrush the tree looks taller': A discourse analysis of men's online groin shaving talk. *Sexualities, 18*(8), 997–1017.

Hall, M., Gough, B., & Hansen, S. (2011). Magazine and reader constructions of 'metrosexuality' and masculinity: A membership categorisation analysis. *Journal of Gender Studies, 20*(1), 69–87.

Hall, M., Gough, B., & Seymour-Smith, S. (2012a). 'I'm METRO, NOT gay', a discursive analysis of men's make-up use on YouTube. *Journal of Men's Studies, 20*(3), 209–226.

Hall, M., Gough, B., & Seymour-Smith, S. (2012b). On-line constructions of metrosexuality and masculinities: A membership categorisation analysis. *Gender and Language, 6*(2), 379–403.

Hall, M., Grogan, S., & Gough, B. (2015). 'It is safe to use if you are healthy': A discursive analysis of men's online accounts of ephedrine use. *Psychology & Health, 30*(7), 770–782.

Hunt, K., Wyke, S., Gray, C. M., Anderson, A. S., Brady, A., Bunn, C., Donnan, P. T., Fenwick, E., Grieve, E., Leishman, J., Miller, E., Mutrie, N., Rauchhaus, P., White, A., & Treweek, S. (2014). A gender-sensitised weight loss and healthy living programme for overweight and obese men delivered by Scottish Premier League football clubs (FFIT): A pragmatic randomised controlled trial. *The Lancet, 383*, 1211–1221.

Immergut, M. (2010). Manscaping: The tangle of nature, culture and male body hair. In L. Moore & M. E. Kosut (Eds.), *The body reader: Essential social and cultural readings* (pp. 287–304). New York: New York University Press.

Jankowski, G. S., Fawkner, H., Slater, A., & Tiggemann, M. (2014). 'Appearance potent'? Are gay men's magazines more "appearance potent" than straight men's magazines in the UK? *Body Image, 11*(4), 474–481.

Jankowski, G., Gough, B., Fawkner, H., Diedrichs, P.C., & Halliwell, E. (submitted). It affects me, it affects me not: The impact of men's body dissatisfaction.

Kanayama, G., Barry, S., Hudson, J. I., & Pope, H. G., Jr. (2006). Body image and attitudes toward male roles in anabolic-androgenic steroid users. *American Journal of Psychiatry, 163*(4), 697–703.

Kehler, M., & Atkinson, M. (Eds.). (2010). *Boys' bodies: Speaking the unspoken.* New York: Peter Lang.

Labre, M. P. (2005). Burn fat, build muscle: A content analysis of men's health and men's fitness. *International Journal of Men's Health, 4*(2), 187–200.

Liossi, C. (2003). *Appearance related concerns across the general and clinical populations.* London: City University. Retrieved from http://ukpmc.ac.uk/theses/ETH/407535

McCormack, M. (2012). *The declining significance of homophobia: How teenage boys are redefining masculinity and heterosexuality.* Oxford/New York: Oxford University Press.

McCreary, D. R., & Sasse, D. K. (2000). An exploration of the drive for muscularity in adolescent boys and girls. *Journal of American College Health, 48,* 297–304.

Mellor, D., Fuller-Tyszkiewicz, M., McCabe, M. P., & Ricciardelli, L. A. (2010). Body image and self-esteem across age and gender: A short-term longitudinal study. *Sex Roles, 63*(9–10), 672–681.

Miller, T. (2005). A metrosexual eye on queer guy. *GLQ: A Journal of Lesbian and Gay Studies, 11,* 112–117.

Miller, T. (2009). *Metrosexuality: See the bright light of commodification shine! Watch yanqui masculinity made over.* Paper presented at the annual meeting of the American Studies Association, 24 May, Accessed 12 May 2010 from http://www.allacademic.com/meta/p105600_index. html

Monaghan, L. F. (2008). Men, physical activity and the obesity discourse: Critical understandings from a qualitative study. *Sociology of Sport Journal: Special Issue on the Social Construction of Fat, 25*(1), 97–128.

Moore, S. (1989). Getting a bit of the other – The pimps of postmodernism. In R. Chapman & J. Rutherford (Eds.), *Male order: Unwrapping masculinity* (pp. 165–192). London: Lawrence & Wishart.

Murray, S., Rieger, E., Touyz, S. W., & De La Garcia, Y. (2010). Muscle dysmorphia and the DSM-V conundrum: Where does it belong? A review paper. *International Journal of Eating Disorders, 43*(6), 483–491.

Olivardia, R., Pope, H. G., Jr., Borowiecki, J. J., & Cohane, G. H. (2004). Biceps and body image: The relationship between muscularity and self-esteem, depression, and eating disorder symptoms. *Psychology of Men & Masculinity, 5*(2), 112–120.

Phoenix, C., & Sparkes, A. C. (2009). Being Fred: Big stories, small stories and the accomplishment of a positive ageing identity. *Qualitative Research, 9*(2), 219–236.

Pope, H. G., Jr., Phillips, K. A., & Olivardia, R. (2000). *The Adonis Complex: The secret crisis of male body obsession.* New York: Free Press.

Ricciardelli, L. A. (2012). Body image development- adolescent boys. In T. Cash (Ed.), *Encyclopedia of body image and human appearance* (pp. 180–187). London: Elsevier.

Ricciardelli, L. A., McCabe, M. P., & Ridge, D. (2006). The construction of the adolescent male body through sport. *Journal of Health Psychology, 11,* 577–587.

Robertson, S. (2006). I've been like a coiled spring this last week': Embodied masculinity and health. *Sociology of Health and Illness, 28*(4), 433–456.

Robertson, S., Sheik, K., & Moore, A. (2010). Embodied masculinities in the context of cardiac rehabilitation. *Sociology of Health & Illness, 32*(5), 695–710.

Roundtree, K. (2005). *A critical sociology of bodybuilding*. Master of Arts Thesis, University of Texas, Arlington.

Sagoe, D., Molde, H., Andreassen, C. S., Torsheim, T., & Pallesen, S. (2014). The global epidemiology of anabolic-androgenic steroid use: A meta-analysis and meta-regression analysis. *Annals of Epidemiology, 24*(5), 383–398.

Seidler, V. J. (1994). *Unreasonable men: Masculinity and social theory*. London: Routledge.

Shilling, C. (1993). *The body and social theory*. London: Sage.

Simpson, M. (1994). *Male impersonators: Men performing masculinity*. London: Cassell.

Simpson, M. (2002). Meet the metrosexual. *Salon*. Retrieved January 4, 2008, from http://dir.salon.com/story/ent/feature/2002/07/22/metrosexual/index2.html

Singleton, P., Fawkner, H.J., White, A., & Foster, S. (2009, October 8). Men's experience of cosmetic surgery: A phenomenological approach to discussion board data. *Qualitative Methods in Psychology Newsletter*, pp. 17–23.

Smith, J. A., & Robertson, S. (2008). Men's health promotion: A new frontier in Australia and the UK? *Health Promotion International, 23*, 283–289.

Smith, D., Rutty, M. C., & Olrich, T. W. (2016). Muscle dysmorphia and anabolic-androgenic steroid use. In M. Hall, S. Grogan, & B. Gough (Eds.), *Chemically modified bodies: The use of substances for appearance enhancement*. Basingstoke: Palgrave.

Stibbe, A. (2004). Health and the social construction of masculinity in Men's health magazine. *Men & Masculinities, 7*, 31–51.

Stice, E., Marti, N. C., Spoor, S., Presnell, K., & Shaw, H. (2008). Dissonance and healthy weight eating disorder prevention programs: Long-term effects from a randomized efficacy trial. *Journal of Consulting and Clinical Psychology, 76*(2), 329–340.

Taylor, N. L. (2011). "Guys, he's humongous!" gender and weight-based teasing in adolescence. *Journal of Adolescent Research, 26*, 178–199.

Watson, J. (2000). *Male bodies: Health, culture and identity*. Buckingham: Open University Press.

CHAPTER 3

Affective Masculinities:
Emotions and Mental Health

Abstract This chapter explores how men today are developing their emotional repertoires, with particular reference to mental health and well-being. Background information on male mental health is provided, relating to men's relative reluctance to seek help for psychological problems, 'masked' depression, and male suicide. Three studies are then featured which focus on how men perform emotions in online environments in situations where they may experience vulnerability: weight management, infertility, and depression. Within these online forums, which offer anonymity and peer support, we witness a range of emotional displays from men, which bodes well for psychological well-being. However, I also note the continued influence of traditional masculinity norms which may operate to constrain, police, or downplay expressions of vulnerability. Implications for male mental health promotion are discussed.

Keywords Emotion • Mental health • Well-being • Vulnerability • Depression

Emotion, or 'affect', has become a focus for social-psychological and sociological analysis and debate in recent years (e.g. Robertson and Monaghan 2012; Wetherell 2012; Burkitt 2002), including in relation to gender and masculinity (e.g. de Boise and Hearn 2017; Lomas et al. 2016; Pease 2012). Sociologists emphasise how privileged men have exercised power

© The Author(s) 2018
B. Gough, *Contemporary Masculinities*,
https://doi.org/10.1007/978-3-319-78819-7_3

over women and other men through the control of emotions (e.g. Seidler 2007; Connell 1995). In fact, emotional control has been valued as a traditional marker of masculinity and promoted within society more generally, for example in workplaces, sport settings, and educational contexts. Traditionally, masculinity norms have promoted rationality, self-reliance, and stoicism, with the realm of emotion disbarred, delegated to women, and coded as weakness or irrationality—except for specific emotions such as anger which are considered more 'masculine' (e.g. Wilkins 2010). This is not to say that men do not *experience* a range of emotions; simply, they have not been encouraged to express feelings or display vulnerability (e.g. Addis and Mahalik 2003).

However, contemporary society now prioritises emotional intelligence, soft skills, and emotional labour across different sites, including personal relationships, workplace interactions, and family life. It is no longer plausible for many men to opt out of emotional expressivity when their partners, children, and clients demand it. Many jobs, for example, increasingly require employees to connect emotionally with colleagues, clients, and stakeholders within service sector industries, from marketing and retail to health and education (see Walker and Roberts 2017)—often impacting negatively on the health and well-being of men from working-class communities (Robertson et al. 2017). In addition, heterosexual relationships constitute a site where men are expected to do emotion. These recent expectations for men clearly clash with more conventional codes of masculinity where emotional suppression is prized, so how do men navigate between these diverse, contradictory injunctions, between 'boys don't cry' and 'it's good to talk'? (McQueen 2017). This chapter attempts to flesh out how men 'do' emotion in relation to different issues—weight management, infertility, and mental health—considering how masculinity is made relevant in such environments. The chapter will conclude by discussing implications for changing masculinities and improving men's emotional well-being.

As noted above, discussions about men and emotion typically suggest that men avoid or suppress emotions apart from anger and aggression. Male stereotypes reinforce such thinking, including the 'strong silent type', the action hero, the absent-minded scientist, and the computer geek, prioritising activity, achievement, and prowess over emotional openness and communication. Such tropes have been dominant for so long and point to a societal privileging of rationality over emotion, action over talk, and attainment over experience. In psychoanalytic terms, men repress their emotions and project them onto women, where they are identified and critiqued (as weak, irrational, excessive), reinforcing sex difference discourse and male power (e.g. Clare 2000).

Despite the traditional idealisation of unemotional men, however, it is increasingly recognised that this stoic norm is not good for men—or their significant others. This point is perhaps most starkly underlined by mental health statistics and trends. In particular, it is now well known that approximately 75% of suicides are committed by men (e.g. ONS 2017). We also know that male depression and anxiety is under-diagnosed (Richards and Borglin 2011), suggesting that many men are reluctant to admit vulnerability and seek help (Addis and Mahalik 2003). When men get distressed, they may exhibit and deal with this indirectly, for example through anger and aggression or alcohol and drug abuse (Brownhill et al. 2005; Addis 2008; Oliffe et al. 2012). This evidence would suggest that male mental health problems are often 'masked' or hidden (Addis 2008). If and when men do seek help for emotional and psychological issues, it is often late in the process when there is a crisis point (e.g. Davidson and Meadows 2010; Johnson et al. 2012). And when men do consult health professionals, they may be faced with advice and treatment which actually reinforces conventional masculine ideals of stoicism and self-discipline (Hale et al. 2010). Outside of medical settings, similar stereotypes may be upheld when men seek help for emotional problems; for example, help-seeking letters submitted to 'experts' within male-targeted magazines found that responses often positioned the men in question in terms of compromised, failed, or insufficient masculinity (Anstiss and Lyons 2014). So, the positioning of men as unemotional (or angry) is widely reproduced—by individual men, by medicine, and by the media. However, that is not to say that (some) men do not express a range of emotions or seek support for psychological issues.

Doing Emotion with Masculinity in Mind

What we have found is that when men feel comfortable with the environment and people around them they are more likely to engage in emotional disclosure. For example, our research on a range of emotionally sensitive topics such as infertility, depression, and weight management demonstrates that many men are happy to share their experiences and emotions online, anonymously (e.g. Hanna and Gough 2016). Clearly, the internet may provide safe spaces for men to open up without revealing their identity or undermining their sense of masculinity. Similarly, McQueen (2017) has found that the men she interviewed were invested in performing emotions in the context of their intimate relationships while being careful not to become too emotional. Likewise, fathering may provide opportunities for many men to expand their repertoire of emotional communication, while distancing themselves from a mothering or feminised position (Hanlon 2012; Hunter et al. 2017). In the workplace, dominated by a service sector requiring social, emotional, and communication skills, men are increasingly compelled towards emotional labour and can adopt various strategies which both underline and resist conventional masculinities (see Lupton 2000). In short, more men are doing emotions across different contexts while navigating between different and sometimes conflicting ideals of masculinity and often taking care to differentiate themselves from women and femininity.

If we return to the arena of mental health and emotional well-being, we find that when men display emotions or seek help for personal problems, they do so when the masculinity conditions are right or can be suitably adjusted. For example, if a man is deemed sufficiently masculine already, that is, has acquired sufficient 'masculine capital' (de Visser et al. 2009), then expressing vulnerability or requesting emotional support may be enabled. In other words, masculine identity will not be threatened by moving into feminised practices if it is already well established. For example, being recognised as an effective soldier may well elicit support from military peers when experiencing distress and seeking help (Green et al. 2010). Other qualitative studies have found that help-seeking may be reframed in masculine ways—men may position themselves or be positioned by others as brave, strong, or even heroic for coming forward. A study by Noone and Stephens (2008), for example, found that older men construed themselves as 'legitimate users' of health services—in contrast to women who were positioned as frequent and trivial attenders, and to other men who did not use services, positioned as naïve or ignorant. In this way, help-seeking is equated with control, rationality, and agency rather than weakness, or even as the pursuit of action and achievement (Johnson et al. 2012). Effectively, it is rational to be emotional. Alternatively, help-seeking may be framed as a means of protecting or advancing valued masculinised roles and capacities, including occupational, familial, and educational responsibilities. For example, Kim et al. (2001) found that some Asian men were more likely to seek help if academic achievement, a greatly cherished objective, was under threat.

Another study reported that older men justified seeking help when it related to sexual functioning, an important identity-relevant practice (Calasanti et al. 2013).

Often, men's relationship to emotions and mental health may oscillate between different enactments and ideals of masculinity. For example, an interview study by Valkonen and Hänninen (2012) focused on men with depression in Finland and suggested that depression could be understood as a consequence of both achieved and unattained hegemonic masculinity—but also that men could both challenge and utilise hegemonic norms as a resource for coping with mental distress. Similarly, Oliffe et al. (2011) interviewed 26 couples where the men self-identified as having depression. They identified three patterns of coping: 'trading places', where the couples exchanged certain stereotypical roles (such as the breadwinner role); 'business as usual', where couples strived to maintain stereotypical roles and thereby conceal any possible 'depression-induced deficits'; and 'edgy tensions', where there was disharmony and/or disagreement in relation to expected roles leading to resentment and threats to sustaining the relationship. To this extent, men's depression is obviously more than an individual experience; rather it is influenced by a range of intersubjective encounters. Another study by Galasinski (2008) based on interviews with depressed men highlighted 'success' stories, where elements of hegemonic masculinity were utilised within these narratives to present a positive male identity despite depression (or even in order to help defeat or control the depression), and stories of 'failure', where the men's suffering was exacerbated by a perceived falling short in relation to masculine norms. Clearly, various elements of masculinity can be negotiated in different ways in efforts to manage emotions and depression.

To examine the phenomenon of men, masculinities, and emotion further, we can consider how men do emotion online across different settings: weight management; infertility; and depression.

ONLINE EMOTION WORK BY MEN

As noted above, it is not that men do not feel or express emotions—they increasingly do so, but in situations where they feel safe and their sense of masculinity is not unduly threatened. In the last chapter we saw that men may use digital spaces and communities (e.g. online discussion forums) to present non-traditional ideals and practices, such as wearing make-up (Hall et al. 2012a, b). More generally, online environments can offer opportunities for self-expression, peer support, and community building (e.g. Paechter 2003). In participating in online interactions with similar others, men may feel free to present emotions (anonymously) without fear of judgement, ridicule, or emasculation. In our projects concerning men's identity work in online communities, we have indeed noted many instances of male emoting, which we will now illustrate with respect to three main topics: weight management, infertility, and depression.

Men and Weight Management

In 2013 we (Bennett and Gough 2013) published a paper based on a study of how men talk to each other about their weight management efforts in an online support group linked to a popular male-targeted magazine. The study can be contextualised with respect to the contemporary explosion in online support groups, encompassing a whole range of health-related topics (see Sullivan 2003, 2008). Although we know that conventional weight loss groups and the concept of 'dieting' are unattractive to most men (Bye et al. 2005; Wilkins 2007), little is known about how all-male group settings might impact on men's weight loss projects, or indeed how men might experience their body size and weight or support each other as they negotiate challenges in this (and other) health-related domain(s). Of interest here is Grogan's (2008) observation that men are increasingly sensitive to body image, more susceptible to bodily dissatisfaction, and more likely to engage in appearance-related practices than previous generations of men. The role of popular culture and mass media in manufacturing fantasies and anxieties around male embodiment, including specific and significant body parts such as the penis, was highlighted by Bordo as early as 1999 in a follow-up to her groundbreaking text on the cultural construction of female bodies and disorders (Bordo 1993). The desire for slender, tight bodies experienced by men and women is firmly situated in culture rather than nature, and amplified in particular mediated contexts such as advertisements in gender-targeted magazines. In light of the contemporary Western emphasis on body projects (Giddens 1991), and given that overweight and obese individuals are widely criticised in contemporary psycho-medical discourse (see Monaghan 2007), it is likely that men who join and contribute to a discussion forum on weight control have to some extent declared their bodies to be problematic. This is not to ignore associations between largesse and hegemonic notions of masculinity, founded on physical presence and occupying space, for example in American football (Pronger 1999) and hip hop culture (Gross 2005), and also in gay 'bear' communities where large bodies are eroticised (Gough and Flanders 2009; Monaghan 2005). Nonetheless, the contributors to our online weight loss forum will be oriented to body modification projects and are likely to be invested in health and/or aesthetic discourses.

Our analysis of the online posts indicated that men were concerned to frame their weight management practices in traditionally masculine ways, for example by using technical bodybuilder jargon to describe discrete muscle groups or construing food preparation in scientific or work terms. Notwithstanding this overarching orientation to conventional masculinity norms, there were instances on the forum where some of the men displayed vulnerability:

> *I'm still not brave enough to go back to the really old pictures! My sister was desperate to show me them last night to prove how well I'd done. But to be honest, the thought scares me, and I'm not lacking motivation at the moment. Those pictures have such an effect on me. I get angry, I have cried looking at them. So it would be a whole load of heartache for not much gain at all really.* (Richy 6, thread 1)

Such reference to feminised emotional phenomena such as 'crying' and 'heartache' and being 'scared' recalls Watson's (2000) experiential embodiment category and was unusual in the forum context. Perhaps the anonymity occasioned by this medium encourages some men to step out of a restricted masculine register, although even in this example there is still some recourse to more traditional 'manly' concepts such as bravery, anger, and pragmatism (reviewing the old photographs is deemed counterproductive). In response to the few instances of such emotional discourse, other contributors produced supportive but concise replies, ranging from the empathetic ('I understand what your saying mate') to the privileging of manly pride over emotional pain ('sod the heartbreak man you should be proud of what you are doing'). This second reply was more typical, highlighting discomfort with and dismissal of feminised emotions, vividly illustrated in this next extract:

> *Loosing weight is not hard stop moaning and get to it. I think you need to read back this post my friend and see how far you have come. Any way enough of this girly stuff.* (Woodie, thread 1)

This post is interesting since support is offered while reaffirming a masculine way of dealing with weight problems. Being emotional is here constructed as a risk to other overweight men, who may be deterred by 'moaning', with the target of the message positioned as a role model. Emotional language is implicitly critiqued as self-centred, neglecting the potential impact on other vulnerable men, and then ultimately and explicitly decried as excessive and feminine ('enough of this girly stuff'). By contrast, action and achievement are elevated ('this guy can do it'; 'get to it') and viewed as 'inspirational'. The focus is certainly on problem- and action-orientated coping.

Men and Infertility

Since 2015 myself and colleague Esmee Hanna have been researching men's accounts of infertility, an issue which affects 1 in 6 couples within the UK (Oakley 2011). Much of the literature in this area focuses on women's experiences (Barnes 2014; Culley et al. 2013), and when men have been included, it has often been as part of a couple, with women's perspectives being the main focus (e.g. Throsby and Gill 2004; Cudmore 2005). There have been some qualitative studies featuring men but not many. One notable study by Malik and Coulson (2008) which looked at men's online accounts highlighted that men perceived their role in terms of supporting their partners while feeling neglected by health professionals given the female focus of clinical approaches to assisting reproduction. As well as being a 'rock' for their partners, men may feel emasculated by their inability to conceive (Barnes 2014). Given the potentially traumatic impact of infertility, we wanted to find out more about how men expressed and negotiated the difficult emotions provoked by infertility—and more broadly to understand the place of emotion in contemporary masculinities.

To access men's accounts of infertility, we (Hanna and Gough 2016) followed Malik and Coulson's (2008) lead and went digital. We found online discussion forums focusing on infertility, with some of these badged as men-only or male-focused. When we looked closely at the discussions, we encountered a lot of emotional 'talk', for example:

> *I constantly get jealous, angry and upset feelings constantly and I like you bite my tongue when some insensitive git starts rambling about the trauma of pregnancy, the sleepless nights and the sick of there [sic] beautiful baby. But I do lose*

my temper and I lose it a lot but I hate myself for feeling this way as I believe that I have no right to think that I deserve a baby more than the next person. (FP5 – Forum Poster 5)

Clearly, strong and complex feelings are engendered by experiences of infertility, which could prove difficult to manage at times, with several men using the phrase 'emotional rollercoaster'. An important factor acknowledged by the men which helped to enable this emotional expressivity was the anonymity provided by the online space:

Thanks for your PM [Private Message]. I do appreciate it, although on this occasion I'm not going to respond, since I do want to keep the anonymity which this site allows. (FP8)

To be identifiable, then, is to risk censure, suggesting that traditional masculinity norms may well inhibit emotional disclosure offline. Indeed, several forum contributors explicitly referenced masculinity constraints:

I know that as men we have an inability to express our feelings but this site has really helped me to come to terms with all the things that are going off in my life. (FP5)

It is somewhat ironic that this stereotype of men's emotional incompetence is voiced in a forum where men are actually expressing a range of difficult emotions—an irony which the men themselves noted. Again, the oscillation between emotional openness and wariness highlights the coexistence of competing masculinities which the men here are attempting to navigate together. Another such indication is the tendency to monitor and dilute emotional content:

It's not counselling or psychiatry, it's just getting it off your chest. (FP2)

There are a lot of people who read here but don't post, so its nice to have someone else joining in, and hopefully we can help if there's anything that you want to get off your chest. (FP8)

In using the phrase 'getting things off your chest', a 'masculine' form of emoting is constructed—differentiated from more formal psychological approaches (i.e. counselling or psychiatry) which may be viewed as feminised (Karepova 2010; Morison et al. 2014). The language used words which minimised the enactment of emotion ('it's just'), attempting to show that the forum is not excessive in terms of its emoting or formalisation.

Men and Depression

As noted earlier, men's seeming reluctance to access psychological services relative to women has been linked to traditional masculinity norms, where displaying vulnerability is construed as weakness. Men suffering from common mental health problems such as depression and anxiety may feel inhibited in revealing their feelings to others, preferring to self-manage (and self-medicate). However, as we have seen above, men can and do present with difficult emotions online, protected by anonymity and encouraged by supportive peers. There are now a number of mental health websites and forums which promote discussion of mental health issues, some of which are tailored to men. With this in mind, I conducted a study exploring how men with depression constructed their illness narratives (Gough 2016). For context, the forum I focused on was linked to a popular men's health magazine which promoted a very action-orientated approach to health and lifestyle issues, positioning men as rational actors with the power to shape and control their bodies, minds, and habits.

What was immediately striking about the men's accounts of their depression was a tendency to reference a diagnosis, as if medical authority was required to legitimise their emotions. Often, a list of symptoms was delineated, with emotional dimensions understated and physical effects foregrounded:

> *my symptoms which were loss of appetite, confidence, heart palpitations, unable to sleep, tearful, and so forth* [T2.1: Thread 2, first post]

Some posts did mention anger and aggression as well as alcohol abuse, but mostly a range of embodied impacts were presented. In discussing medication, most men on the forum portrayed this as a necessarily evil, a forced, temporary choice at odds with a preference for self-management:

> *a course of antidepressants just to get myself back on the track … I'm aware they won't solve all my problems, but merely getting me mentally back into a state where I want to work out, get up in the morning and generally operate on a basic level would be great, a means to an end.* [T23.1]

Being in control of feelings and behaviour was paramount for many men.

For those men who had not (yet) received a diagnosis, the task for them was to construct a plausible account of their depression, that is one which was not too emotional (since action is valued in this community) or subjective (since only doctors are qualified to diagnose). Hence, in their depression stories men emphasised their own efforts to deal with it themselves—mirroring the ethos of the magazine:

I am determined to get through this. I have been doing my very best to get out and see people, offload and keep busy, but it's not enough to get me out of this hole. [T2.1]

So, what we witness here is a construction of self as actively combatting depression as far as possible while recognising the difficulty of succeeding. In this way, the men were able to avoid possible implications of personal weakness or blame for their distress. Other strategies for managing this accountability included drawing attention to extenuating circumstances (e.g. bereavement, job loss, divorce) and emphasising the destructive behaviour of significant others (e.g. ex-partner terminating the relationship). Overall, then, the contributors to the forum were minded to privilege bodily impacts over feelings in their depression stories, and action-based remedies over psychological or pharmacological intervention. It is clear that in this magazine-linked context traditional masculinity norms operate to constrain the expression of emotions within accounts of depression and its management.

IMPLICATIONS

As indicated above, it would be a mistake to think men lack in emotion or are disinclined to share their feelings. Recent research suggests that men do express a range of emotions—when the environment is deemed safe, supportive, and 'male-friendly'. The presentation of emotions is not straightforward, however, with many men seemingly influenced by traditional masculinity norms, which prompt them to downplay, police, or otherwise 'masculinise' emotional talk.

Arguably, current mental health service provision could be more 'male-friendly'. It has been noted, for example, that the majority of counsellors, therapists, and clinical psychologists are female—which may be one factor which discourages some men from seeking professional help (see Morison et al. 2014). Given that men's depression may be 'masked' (Addis 2008), when men actually do access services their symptoms may be misread and mistreated since their distress presentation may well veer from standard checklists (e.g. violence, alcohol abuse, psychosomatic gastric problems, etc.; Wilkins 2010). In addition, the traditional focus on emotion talk within therapeutic settings may discourage some men—men may prefer to focus on thoughts rather than dwelling on feelings, so cognitive (e.g. cognitive-behavioural therapy [CBT]) and mindfulness (Lomas 2014) interventions may be attractive. Another advantage of CBT for men is its pragmatic, problem-solving focus—an instrumental coping style that men supposedly favour (Lazarus and Folkman 1984; Robertson 2007).

In efforts to engage more men, some mental health promotion campaigns have invoked masculinity norms. For example, help-seeking can be reframed in terms of toughness and independence, while marketing discourse and imagery may invoke sport, war, or work references (see Samaritans 2012). Similarly, community-based initiatives have marketed their programmes carefully, for example avoiding clinical language and foregrounding particular activities such as sport, do it yourself (DIY), and information technology (IT) sessions. A well-established programme targeting mainly older, isolated men is the Men's Sheds initiative, which promotes men making things together which may then be used in their communities. The UK Men's Sheds Association (www.menssheds.org.uk) states that there are now over 80 Sheds in the UK. Such initiatives characterise a 'shoulder-to-shoulder' rather than 'face-to-face' approach where men do emotion indirectly, side by side, in the context of another activity (see Robertson 2007). Many of these programmes build in social space and time where men can enjoy each other's company, learn to trust others, and gradually work through any problems they may be experiencing.

Some men's mental health promotions have prioritised sport; for example, It's a Goal (www.itsagoal.org.uk) is an 11-week therapeutic programme based at football venues which uses football metaphors to reach men with mental health needs. Similarly, Time to Change (www.time-to-change.org.uk/), the UK anti-stigma mental health campaign, has used football metaphors in resources aimed at encouraging men to talk about mental health problems. Leaflets and 'top tips' cards are branded 'Is your mate off his game? … Get on the ball about mental health'. Another initiative draws on boxing metaphors and images ('be in your mate's corner'). These and other programmes also deploy humour in sessions and resources in order to encourage men to talk to their friends about mental health problems.

These community programmes vary in terms of professional and peer input. In some cases, professional psychological input may be available or advertised within the community space, while in others the focus is very much on peer support. Peers may be trained by professionals and are well placed to refer men to other services, and if peer facilitators hail from the same community then they are more likely to be respected and responded to. In general, the more a service can be designed, developed, and delivered with community members from the start, where local values, language, and facilities are central, the more are the chances of community buy-in and success (see Robertson et al. 2013).

Clearly, online communities can serve to encourage men to open up and receive support. Recent mental health initiatives in different countries have attempted to engage men in just this way. For example, Campaign Against Living Miserably (CALM) in the UK provides a web chat service, with text and online options, especially popular with younger men, who may start with text, then move to talking on the phone. CALM also displays a marked preference for non-medical language—'feeling shit' rather than 'being depressed'—and uses musicians and actors as ambassadors to communicate with men without expecting them to adhere to a script or use clinical language. With such programmes there is a balance to be struck between invoking strengths-based masculine ideals and challenging some of the more restrictive aspects of masculinity. In Canada, the men's depression 'help yourself' website (http://www.mensdepressionhelpyourself.ubc.ca/) showcases the findings drawn from a programme of research on masculinities and men's depression. Focused on college, middle-aged, and older men, content is targeted to specific age groups amid offering guidance about men's depression through video vignettes drawn from men experiencing depression and health-care providers who treat men's depression.

Other organisations are testing such remote, anonymous forms of support for men. For example, Relate (www.relate.org.uk) provides telephone counselling, email counselling, and live online chat. Online provision can range from discussion forums and support groups involving peers to email and messaging forms of counselling. Websites and online resources are hosted by a range of non-governmental organisations (NGOs) and may be general (e.g. menshealthforum.org) or address a particular problem or constituency (e.g. mengeteatingdisorderstoo.co.uk).

In sum, we are now witnessing greater facilitation of men's emotional expression across mental health and community (including online) contexts. Arguably, more men are now more amenable to engage emotionally when they feel comfortable and encouraged, whether with peers or professionals. The importance of traditional masculinity norms remains, however—as men negotiate emotions within diverse contexts they often take care to manage their disclosures carefully, as well of those of peers.

REFERENCES

Addis, M. E. (2008). Gender and depression in men. *Clinical Psychology: Science and Practice, 15,* 153–168.

Addis, M. E., & Mahalik, J. (2003). Men, masculinity and the contexts of help seeking. *American Psychologist, 58*(1), 5–14.

Anstiss, D., & Lyons, A. (2014). From men to the media and back again: Help-seeking in popular men's magazines. *Journal of Health Psychology, 19*(11), 1358–1370.

Barnes, L. (2014). *Conceiving masculinity: Male infertility, medicine, and identity.* Philadelphia: Temple University Press.

Bennett, E., & Gough, B. (2013). In pursuit of leanness: Constructing bodies and masculinities online within a men's weight management forum. *Health, 17*(3), 284–299.

Bordo, S. (1993). *Unbearable weight: Feminism, western culture and the body.* Berkeley: University of California Press.

Brownhill, S., Wilhelm, K., Barclay, L., & Schmied, V. (2005). 'Big Build': hidden depression in men. *Australian and New Zealand Journal of Psychiatry, 39*(10), 921–931.

Burkitt, I. (2002). Complex emotions: Relations, feelings and images in emotional experience. *The Sociological Review, 50*(S2), 151–167.

Bye, C., Avery, A., & Lavin, J. (2005). Tackling obesity in men - preliminary evaluation of men only groups within a commercial slimming organization. *Journal of Human Nutrition and Dietetics, 18,* 391–394.

Calasanti, T., Pietila, I., Ojala, H., & King, N. (2013). Men, bodily control, and health behaviours: The importance of age. *Health Psychology, 32*(1), 15–23.

Clare, A. (2000). *On men: Masculinity in crisis.* London: Chatto and Windus.

Connell, R. W. (1995). *Masculinities.* Cambridge: Polity Press.

Cudmore, L. (2005). Becoming parents in the context of loss. *Sexual and Relationship Therapy, 20,* 299–308.

Culley, L., Hudson, N., & Hohan, M. (2013). Where are all the men? The marginalization of men in social scientific research on infertility. *Reproductive Biomedicine Online, 27,* 225–235.

Davidson, K., & Meadows, R. (2010). Older men's health: The role of marital status and masculinities. In B. Gough & S. Robertson (Eds.), *Men, masculinities & health: Critical* (pp. 109–124). Basingstoke: Palgrave.

De Boise, S., & Hearn, J. (2017). Are men getting more emotional? Critical sociological perspectives on men, masculinities and emotion. *The Sociological Review,* 1–18.

de Visser, R. O., Smith, J. A., & McDonnell, E. J. (2009). 'That's not masculine': Masculine capital and health-related behaviour. *Journal of Health Psychology, 14*(7), 1047–1058.

Galasinski, D. (2008). *Men's discourses of depression.* Basingstoke: Palgrave.

Giddens, A. (1991). *Modernity and self-identity: Self and society in the late modern age.* Cambridge: Polity Press.

Gough, B. (2016). Men's depression talk online: A qualitative analysis of accountability and authenticity in help-seeking and support formulations. *Psychology of Men & Masculinity, 17,* 156–165.

Gough, B., & Flanders, G. (2009). Celebrating 'Obese' bodies: Gay 'Bears' talk about weight, body image and health. *International Journal of Men's Health, 8*(3), 235–253.

Green, G., Emslie, C., O'Neill, D., Hunt, K., & Walker, S. (2010). Exploring the ambiguities of masculinity in accounts of emotional distress in the military among ex-servicemen. *Social Science & Medicine, 71*(8), 1480–1488.

Grogan, S. (2008). *Body image: Understanding body dissatisfaction in men, women, and children.* London: Routledge.

Gross, J. (2005). Phat. In D. Kulick & A. Meneley (Eds.), *Fat: The anthropology of an obsession* (pp. 63–76). New York: Penguin.

Hale, S., Grogan, S., & Willott, S. (2010). Male GPs' views on men seeking medical help: A qualitative study. *British Journal of Health Psychology, 15*(4), 697–713.

Hall, M., Gough, B., & Seymour-Smith, S. (2012a). 'I'm METRO, NOT gay', a discursive analysis of men's make-up use on YouTube. *Journal of Men's Studies, 20*(3), 209–226.

Hall, M., Gough, B., & Seymour-Smith, S. (2012b). On-line constructions of metrosexuality and masculinities: A membership categorisation analysis. *Gender and Language, 6*(2), 379–403.

Hanlon, N. (2012). *Masculinities, care and equality: Identity and nurture in men's lives.* Basingstoke: Palgrave.

Hanna, E., & Gough, B. (2016). Emoting infertility online: A qualitative analysis of men's forum posts. *Health, 20*(4), 363–382.

Hunter, C., Riggs, D. W., & Augoustinos, M. (2017). Constructions of primary caregiving fathers in popular parenting texts. *Men and Masculinities.* https://doi.org/10.1177/1097184X17730593.

Johnson, J. L., Oliffe, J. L., Kelly, M. T., Galdas, P., & Ogrodniczuk, J. S. (2012). Men's discourses of help-seeking in the context of depression. *Sociology of Health & Illness, 34,* 345–361.

Karepova, M. (2010). *Psychological counselling in Russia: The making of a feminised profession.* PhD Thesis, University of York, UK.

Kim, B. S., Atkinson, D. R., & Umemoto, D. (2001). Asian cultural values and the counseling process: Current knowledge and directions for future research. *The Counseling Psychologist, 29*(4), 570–603.

Lazarus, R. S., & Folkman, S. (1984). *Stress, appraisal and coping*. New York: Springer.

Lomas, T. (2014). *Masculinity, meditation, and mental health*. Basingstoke: Palgrave.

Lomas, T., Cartwright, T., Edginton, T., & Ridge, D. (2016). New ways of being a man: Positive hegemonic masculinity in meditation-based communities of practice. *Men and Masculinities, 19*, 289–310.

Lupton, B. (2000). Maintaining masculinity: Men who do women's work. *British Journal of Management, 11*(S1), 33–48.

Malik, A., & Coulson, N. (2008). The male experience of infertility: A thematic analysis of an online infertility support group bulletin board. *Journal of Reproductive and Infant Psychology, 26*, 18–30.

McQueen, F. (2017). Male emotionality: 'Boys don't cry' versus 'it's good to talk'. *NORMA: International Journal for Masculinity Studies, 12*(3–4). https://doi.org/10.1080/18902138.2017.1336877.

Monaghan, L. F. (2005). Big handsome men, bears and others: Virtual constructions of 'fat male embodiment'. *Body & Society, 11*(2), 81–111.

Monaghan, L. F. (2007). Body mass index, masculinities and moral worth: Men's critical understandings of 'appropriate' weight-for-health. *Sociology of Health & Illness, 29*(4), 584–609.

Morison, L., Trigeorgis, C., & John, M. (2014). Are mental health services inherently feminised? *The Psychologist, 27*, 414–417.

Noone, J. H., & Stephens, C. (2008). Men, masculine idendities, and health care utilisation. *Sociology of Health & Illness, 30*(5), 711–725.

Oakley, L. (2011). *The epidemiology of infertility: Measurement, prevalence and an investigation of early life and reproductive, risk factors*. PhD Thesis, London School of Hygiene and Tropical Medicine. Available at: http://researchonline.lshtm.ac.uk/682432/1/549753.pdf. Accessed 17 Sept 2015.

Oliffe, J. L., Han, C. S., Ogrodniczuk, J. S., Phillips, J. C., & Roy, P. (2011). Suicide from the perspectives of older men who experience depression: A gender analysis. *American Journal of Men's Health, 5*, 444–454.

Oliffe, J., Ogrodniczuk, J. S., Bottorff, J. L., Johnson, J. L., & Hoyak, K. (2012). 'You feel like you can't live anymore': Suicide from the perspectives of Canadian men who experience depression. *Social Science & Medicine, 74*(4), 506–514.

ONS. (2017). *Suicides in the UK: 2016 registrations*. London: Office for National Statistics.

Paechter, C. (2003). Masculinities and feminities as communities of practice. *Women's Studies International Forum, 26*(1), 69–77.

Pease, B. (2012). The politics of gendered emotions: Disrupting men's emotional investment in privilege. *Australian Journal of Social Issues, 47*, 125–142.

Pronger, B. (1999). Outta my endzone: Sport and the territorial anus. *Journal of Sport and Social Issues, 23*, 373–389.

Richards, D. A., & Borglin, G. (2011). Implementation of psychological therapies for anxiety and depression in routine practice: Two year prospective cohort study. *Journal of Affective Disorders, 133*, 51–60.

Robertson, S. (2007). *Understanding men and health: Masculinities, identity and well-being.* Buckingham: Open University Press.

Robertson, S., & Monaghan, L. (2012). Embodied heterosexual masculinities part 2: Foregrounding Men's health and emotions. *Sociology Compass, 6*(2), 151–165.

Robertson, S., Witty, K., Zwolinsky, S., & Day, R. (2013). Men's health promotion interventions: What have we learned from previous programmes? *Community Practitioner, 86*(11), 38–41.

Robertson, S., Gough, B., & Robinson, M. (2017). Masculinities and health inequalities within neoliberal economies. In C. Walker & S. Roberts (Eds.), *Masculinity, labour, and neoliberalism: Working-class men in international perspective.* Basingstoke: Palgrave Macmillan.

Samaritans. (2012). *Men, suicide and society. Research report.* www.samaritans.org

Seidler, V. (2007). Masculinities, bodies, and emotional life. *Men and Masculinities, 10*, 9–21.

Sullivan, C. F. (2003). Gendered cybersupport: A thematic analysis of two online cancer support groups. *Journal of Health Psychology, 8*(1), 83–103.

Sullivan, C. F. (2008). Cybersupport: Empowering asthma caregivers. *Pediatric Nursing, 34*(3), 217–224.

Throsby, K., & Gill, R. (2004). It's different for men: Masculinity and IVF. *Men & Masculinities, 6*, 330–348.

Valkonen, J., & Hänninen, V. (2012). Narratives of masculinity and depression. *Men & Masculinities, 16*(2), 160–180.

Walker, C., & Roberts, S. (Eds.). (2017). *Masculinity, labour and neoliberalism: Working class men in international perspective.* Basingstoke: Palgrave.

Watson, J. (2000). *Male bodies: Health, culture and identity.* Buckingham: Open University Press.

Wetherell, M. (2012). *Affect and emotion: A new social science understanding.* London: Sage.

Wilkins, D. (2007). The research base for male obesity: What do we know? In A. White & M. Pettifer (Eds.), *Hazardous waist: Tackling male weight problems* (pp. 3–11). Abingdon: Radcliffe Publishing.

Wilkins, D. (2010). *Untold problems: A review of the essential issues in the mental health of men and boys.* London: Men's Health Forum.

CHAPTER 4

Supportive Masculinities: Caring for Others

Abstract This chapter explores men's caring practices across different settings, ranging from offering support to peers online or in the pub to nurturing children and becoming allies to women and gay men. Literature on 'caring masculinities' stems mainly from studies of fatherhood and this work is summarised to set the scene. Three extended research examples of caring masculinities are then presented: firstly, examining how men experiencing infertility provide support and guidance to peers in fraternal ways within online forums; then, looking at how involved and stay-at-home fathers report on their experiences in gendered ways; lastly, highlighting accounts of men who have volunteered to work with organisations committed to supporting equality and combating sexism and homophobia. Implications for changing masculinities—and social change—are discussed.

Keywords Care • Peer support • Fatherhood • Allies • Social change

Traditionally, men support each other indirectly, shoulder to shoulder, through actions more than words (e.g. Robertson 2007). Media discourses pertaining to advice and support for men reinforce traditional masculinities, for example within male-targeted magazines (e.g. Anstiss and Lyons 2014). Similarly, men have been conventionally defined outwith the home, positioned as breadwinners and strong silent types who

© The Author(s) 2018
B. Gough, *Contemporary Masculinities*,
https://doi.org/10.1007/978-3-319-78819-7_4

support their partners and families through working, providing resources, and being strong (e.g. Dolan 2007). Now, in tandem with expanding repertoires of emotional expression and body projects, men are increasingly getting involved in supporting and caring for others, whether it is peers with shared experiences, family members, or other groups (e.g. women or lesbian, gay, bisexual, transgender, queer [LGBTQ]) seeking justice and equality.

The research we have done examining men's contributions to various online community forums highlights many instances of providing support to other men, ranging from positive endorsements of cosmetic practices to sympathy and practical advice offered to men experiencing infertility or depression. While there is often a self-conscious or muted delivery of support, suggesting the continued operation of traditional masculinities which code emotion and nurturance as feminised, this fraternal mode of help-giving is much appreciated by recipients. And, as noted in previous chapters, online environments offer the anonymity which may facilitate caring, and supportive behaviours otherwise absent or under-elaborated offline between men.

Nonetheless, it is noteworthy that men are hugging each other more so than previous generations, at least in some Western nations like the UK, although perhaps not with the same gusto or openness as women. And among younger men, there is some evidence of caring for peers in a range of tactile ways (hugging, cuddling, kissing), leading some to claim a softer, more 'inclusive' masculinity (Anderson 2009), although the evidence is not yet developed (see O'Neill 2015). A 'caring masculinity' has also been applied to contemporary fatherhood practices (Hanlon 2012) and to men's intimate relationships (McQueen 2017). Beyond their immediate communities, there is evidence that more men are getting involved in campaigns and organisations dedicated to diversity, equality, and inclusion—caring for other groups. Work we are conducting with non-governmental organisations (NGOs) such as Sport Allies and the Great Men project has informed us about men's individual and collective interest in and commitment to improving quality of life for women, gay men, and other groups—and men's personal and political development. This chapter will illustrate a range of situations where men are enacting 'supportive masculinities'. Reflecting on these developments, some issues and debates bearing on the opportunities and resources for (some) men to reach out to others will be highlighted.

CONTEMPORARY FATHERHOOD

Perhaps the bulk of research concerned with caring masculinities has focused on fatherhood (e.g. Hanlon 2012). For various reasons, men are increasingly becoming more involved in childcare and family life more generally (e.g. Doucet 2006; Scambor et al. 2014). In many societies it is becoming increasingly untenable for men to opt out of everyday childcare to focus on their careers. Although breadwinning can be considered a form of care, wider social changes (female employment; flexible working; job precarity; gender equality norms, etc.) mean that more men are more involved in childcare today. There is debate about how much caring work men do in practice, with many suggesting that the discourse of the modern involved father is not yet fully enacted on the ground (see Hanlon 2012; Finn and Henwood 2009), a view supported by statistics on gendered distribution of unpaid childcare and housework (e.g. women do 40% more than men on average: ONS 2016). Within every family, men navigate between traditional and modern fatherhood ideals—and diverse masculine positions—with varying displays of care and affection.

In a landmark study, Hanlon (2012) interviewed diverse groups of Irish men about their definitions and negotiations around their fathering/caring practices. He encountered a range of positions and identified three main categories of father: conventionalists—men committed to breadwinning; sharers—men who valued breadwinning and involved fatherhood; and carers—men who were most involved in caring for their children, although usually through circumstances and not by choice. Overall, Hanlon (2012: 203) noted that caring activities encouraged a softer, relational masculinity.

There is also emerging evidence that men frame their childcare differently to women, emphasising 'masculine' aspects (e.g. Robinson et al. 2011; Doucet 2006), such as event management (e.g. family outings: Lynch et al. 2009). In addition, it has been found that male caregivers can find it difficult to seek support because it means admitting vulnerability and they can also have less extensive friendships and care networks to draw from than women. They may also feel it is their responsibility to manage the home situation alone (Weinland 2009; Applegate and Kaye 1993; Fraser and Warr 2009).

The importance of masculinity is also promoted by 'stay-at-home-dads', as a recent study by Hunter et al. (2017) suggests. In this study, various Australian parenting texts authored by male primary caregivers targeting other men were analysed. Here, the authors noticed a preoccupation with masculinity. For example, breadwinning/employment was still regarded as important, something that could be re-engaged in while the children were at school. In addition, masculine credentials earned before the current caregiving role were foregrounded, such as sporting or work achievements. Caring itself was branded in masculine terms:

> *There's no doubt that playtime with Dad is a bit more physical than it is with my wife. I like to get down on my hands and knees and let the kids jump on my back like they're riding a horse. My wife is a bit too dainty to do that and prefers a less rough and tumble playtime when they're together.*

> *Kids need to learn from playing, using their imagination, and even falling down. That's what dads bring to the table.*

> *Expect dads to do things differently from moms. Women ask for directions. Men use tools. Face it, men and women are different, in their parenting styles as well as in other ways, and their differences should be recognised and embraced.*

Here, sex difference discourse is clearly reproduced, with fathering contrasted with mothering. As caregiving is associated with women and femininity, these fathers sought to reframe their practices with reference to traditional masculinity ideals. Beyond the home environment, concerns about masculinity recur where care and support are directed to peers.

PEER SUPPORT

Outside the family, there is some evidence that men, especially younger men, are developing more caring, supportive masculinities in relation to their (male) friends. Anderson (2014: 6) and colleagues argue that younger men today are less homophobic and more affectionate towards each other:

> *They are not afraid to enact their brotherly love to one another, not afraid of being homosexualized by their behaviors. Thus, while they are likely the first generation to never attend a protest, they politic through their Facebook and Twitter accounts. They also take political action against the previous generation's masculinity by engaging in public displays of homosocial affection (same-sex behaviors without sexual attraction).*

Based on several studies conducted by himself and his colleagues, Anderson proposes that young men today kiss, cuddle, and sleep together without fear of judgement. Although this work has been questioned (O'Neill 2015), with criticisms ranging from limited samples to selective, post-feminist theorising, this positive view of heteromasculinity chimes with the thesis that masculinity is evolving and becoming more caring and 'inclusive'. However, how men express love and care for each other varies greatly by context. For example, in some best-selling men's magazines, the repertoire of caring masculinities is limited.

While the men's style press has promoted images of fashion-conscious metrosexual masculinities, the majority of mainstream male-targeted magazines project a more traditional heteronormative ideal centred on lean-muscular bodies, sexual prowess, and personal control (e.g. Stibbe 2004). Advice sought by readers and delivered within the magazine focuses on particular body projects relating to exercise, nutrition, and sexual attraction/performance (Stevenson et al. 2000; Ricciardelli et al. 2010). This narrow repertoire of topics and regimes belies an avoidance of emotions, an editing out of vulnerability and softer notions of masculinity. This traditional discourse of masculinity is reinforced via a number of interlocking discursive strategies, as Anstiss and Lyons (2014) note. In their analysis of the letters and advice provided by magazine experts within two mainstream men's magazines (FHM and Men's Health, four issues each published between November 2009 and February 2010), they identified three main devices. First, they highlight the deployment of technical jargon in relation to body problems, for example:

Question: *I play Aussie rules football and experience sore legs a couple of days after the match. What is the best method of recovery to reduce this – ice bath, a low impact activity or massage?*

Response: *Delayed-onset muscle soreness (DOMS) is very common, and all of your suggestions are probably helpful. Anti-inflammatory tablets reduce DOMS as well. If it is very severe and always in a specific part of your legs, you should get a professional consultation to assess for specific diagnosis (e.g. compartment syndrome of the calves, back related hamstring pain).*

In this extract, both the help-seeker and (especially) the expert display specialist knowledge, use health terms (DOMS), and focus on practical solutions. The role of medicine is promoted via references to medication and medical expertise ('professional consultation' for a 'diagnosis'). It is also interesting that the account of pain is under-elaborated; another feature of the data is an emphasis on pain endurance, for example:

Question: *I've injured my sternum after a chest workout. My GP thinks it's where the rib meets the sternum and that the cartilage is inflamed/damaged. Is there anything you recommend?*

Response: *We see this injury occasionally in sports medicine and it is tough to treat. It's probably a type of stress fracture between the rib cartilage and sternum, which is bone. It's more common in younger athletes when there are extra growth plates around the sternum. Longer term rest may fix it and active stimulatory treatments (ultrasounds and similar machines at the physio) may heal it. The best news is that it shouldn't get worse. If the pain is bearable, you can just train through it.*

In this extract we again observe the use of technical language, but another key theme is the manly tolerance of pain (and the continuation of physical activity)—clearly reproducing a conventional masculine stoicism which eschews vulnerability and prizes strength (training). Away from sporting environments, some body problems/solutions are feminised (and problematised), for example:

Question: *The skin on the back of my hands is dry and painful. Do I need to take a trip to a girly nail parlour or are there some home remedies?*

Response: *Either way, prepare to leave your manhood at the door. 'A good quality manicure will deal with cuticle dryness, as a nail technician will apply a hand moisturiser at the end', says Maria Epiphaniuo, therapist at a trendy bloke's grooming salon. But if you can't bear to leave the house on such a mission, have a go yourself, as Maria explains. 'Use a homemade mask by slightly warming up some olive oil and soaking your hands in it. Follow this by wrapping the hands with cling film, and then wrap them in a damp, hot towel for 10 minutes'. When you're done, why not chop your own gonads off?*

Here the help-seeker and the responder explicitly construct skin interventions as unmasculine ('girly'), a domain where men may be symbolically castrated. This rejection of skincare and grooming clearly contrasts with our data on metrosexual masculinities where, for example, cosmetic use is promoted (albeit still with some reference to conventional masculinities: Hall et al. 2012a, b). Context is obviously crucial—in some (e.g. online) environments help-seeking and care for others can be accomplished with less concern about traditional masculinities than is evident within mainstream male-targeted magazines.

Another site for male support and advice—and the reproduction of traditional masculinities—is the pub. Although drunkenness, fighting, and womanising are conventionally associated with (mainly working-class) men and drinking, pubs have also brought men together and have proved important for identity and well-being (e.g. Gough and Edwards 1998; Peralta 2007). Although most pubs today are welcoming towards women, some men may value such venues as sources of homosocial bonding, a space where difficulties can be forgotten or hinted at, and support can be enjoyed, however indirect. An interesting study by Emslie et al. (2013) explored peer support and well-being within the pub among middle-aged men in Scotland. These men highlighted the role of alcohol as a social 'lubricant', enabling them to 'open up' among friends. They also advocated social drinking as protective against mental health problems, as one participant notes:

CALLUM: *If you go out with your mates, have a few drinks, it's great for your mental health. You don't feel lonely, you don't feel sad or depressed, it always cheers you up, you know. So I'd say that that's a huge benefit. (…) I don't think men can express themselves as well as women. So I think yeah- a lot of time men need-especially young men, I know what the statistic rates are like for men committing suicide in the UK is pretty high, men I think need other people around them. You need your mates, as I said, to keep you sane.* (FG13)

Simply being with male friends in the pub then is associated with benefits to well-being, regardless of any explicit help-seeking or discussion of personal issues. The homosocial pub context was also promoted as a site where friends in trouble could be cared for:

EWAN: *We've got a friend who's gone missing, and we know the best thing for him is to get him out, you know. I've been offering him work to*

> *try and get him out, cause we were worried it was money or what-*
> *ever it is. And we instinctively know his mental health can't be*
> *right. So it's a very important issue and if it's surrounded by*
> *drink there's a problem there, but it's an import- more than a sup-*
> *port mechanism, it's a- to me it's a critical and normal and nat-*
> *ural and welcoming and positive part of life.*

Here, the pub is construed as a sanctuary, an emphatically positive space where friends can be recuperated under the care of their mates. Although it is conceded that alcohol can generate problems, on the whole drinking together with friends is presented as a source of belonging, support, and well-being. In our own work we have found much evidence of men supporting each other in various online environments—arguably in more direct, elaborate ways compared to more traditional male-friendly environments such as men's magazines and pubs.

PEER SUPPORT ONLINE

Our various projects examining how men enact vulnerability and seek support online have provided insights into how such accounts are responded to by peers. What we have witnessed is an outpouring of support, advice, and care within male-only or male-dominated communities online. Displays of support by men online can operate to uphold traditional notions of masculinity and/or more modern versions. For example, in the study of depression talk within an online forum linked to the *Men's Health* magazine (Gough 2016), many responses advocated practical support and self-help strategies:

> *Go to your doctor … lots of exercise, no alcohol, massages, talking about it to*
> *friends/family, breathing techniques.* [T7.2]

> *See a doctor … learn a new sport or start intensive training at the gym.*
> [T15.2]

> *doctors asap … get more hobbies like say sports meet people keep busy.* [T22.2]

> *Go to the doctor … there are other options available to you other than drugs that*
> *also work.* [T23.2]

Although talking about problems is sometimes advocated (e.g., T7.2 above), many more responding posts propose more action-oriented strategies (sport, training, etc.), thereby reinforcing the conventional association of masculinity with the external, physical world rather than the internal, psychological world (Courtenay 2000; Rochlen et al. 2010). However, in other online communities independent of men's magazines, we encounter a softer repertoire, as in our study of how male bodybuilders talk to each other online about synthol—an oil that can be injected into muscles to enhance their size (Hall et al. 2015). In the following extract, painful side effects of synthol injections are normalised:

Original post: *Has anyone else had these muscle pains after their SYNTHOL injections.*
                   please let me know thank you

Response post: *Absolutely normal brother. Also the bruising does occur often with me, but*
                   Synthelamin B-12 calmed it a lot. But yes I did bruise most of the time. The outcome you will be impressed with so just stick with it. Keep your stock up, because with what you are doing you'll want to keep a few bottles on hand. It does go rather quickly for such a large bottle because of the large doses per day. Good luck man.

Here there are echoes of Anstiss and Lyon's (2014) themes around masculine tolerance of pain and practical recommendations in response to queries. In addition, however, the respondent offers reassurance, shares his own experience, and sends good wishes, suggesting a warmer, empathetic masculinity at work within a supportive homosocial community ('brother'; 'good luck man'). We also know that advice and support are greatly appreciated by men within online forums. For example, the provider of the make-up tutorial for men (see Hall et al. 2012a, b) received a lot of praise:

you did great! a+
its nice to see another guy like me who wears makeup.
hey bro good shit im right there wit ya.
nice one !!

These positive endorsements indicate a supportive community, where like-minded men share interests and value peer advice—while still emphasising their masculinity ('guy'; 'bro'). Similarly, men experiencing infertility (see Hanna and Gough 2016) express gratitude for support received from peers:

> *I'm really glad I've found a forum for guys on this rocky road. ... I seem to have spent the last month or two finding endless forums for women to share their conception/fertility woes but nothing for men. ... I have been feeling pretty down about the whole thing and really wanted to find somewhere to chat with other people who had been through it all as you do end up feeling like there isn't anyone you can talk to. (FP1)*

Clearly, online spaces enable many men to offer support and share experiences on a range of issues—and in doing so to [re]construct masculinities with reference to conventional and modern expectations. As noted, doing support can range from providing practical advice centred on self-reliance to exchanging personal stories and sharing emotions. And even in male-dominated sites such as men's magazines and pubs, forms of support are on offer and demonstrate care for other men. Beyond families, friends, and peers, men and boys are increasingly becoming involved in making caring interventions through supporting campaigns and organisations which pursue social change.

Supporting Others: Men as Advocates and Allies

Despite past and present anti-feminist backlashes, men's rights movements, and sexual violence against women, there are historic and more recent examples of men getting involved in feminist struggles and debates about men's role within feminism more generally. Academic work in the field of critical studies of men and masculinities has been important for critiquing dominant (hegemonic) masculinity ideals and their impact on subordinated and marginalised men and women (Connell 1995). More recently, however, the field is starting to explore how men and masculinities can be appropriated for the good of men and women, as in Anderson's (2009) concept of inclusive masculinities or Lomas's (2013) work on 'critically positive masculinity'. Various EU-funded projects have sought to promote the role of men in gender equality, with a key focus on involving men in childcare (e.g. Scambor et al. 2014). It is certainly striking today that there are a range of initiatives which recruit men to support groups experiencing prejudice and discrimination (women; gay men) and to challenge toxic notions of masculinity.

For example, MenEngage (http://menengage.org/) is a global alliance of organisations working with men to promote gender equality and reduce conflict. In the UK, the White Ribbon Campaign seeks to engage men and organisations in challenging violence against women (https://www.whiteribbon.org.uk/).

Another UK initiative, the Great Men Project, recruits male volunteers to deliver workshops with schoolboys in London which are designed to deconstruct traditional masculinity norms. The project website (https://www.great-men.org/portraits) features 'portraits' of volunteers where some write about their motivations and aspirations. For example, Adam writes:

> *If we want a more gender equal society, then we have to start removing the barriers to it. As I see it one of the big barriers is men or – more specifically – the ideas, values and behaviours that society encourages us to associate with being a man. This project seeks to encourage young men to question the kind of men they might feel encouraged to be and get them to ask what kind of men they want to become.*

In conversations with young men at school, dominant masculinities are challenged and alternative ways of being a man imagined. As well as focusing on younger men, the volunteers also recognise their own complicity in perpetuating sexism and the need for themselves as well as others to change:

> *Everyday I witness the accepted degradation of women in which I also have played a part. It's time to express the truth and not hold back, for in staying silent we are complicit to the abuse. The change comes from each of us making a different choice and adding to the groundswell. I got involved with Great Men because it is at the forefront in implementing those changes in a proactive and powerful way – by inspiring the next generation who have the potential to be Great men.* (Jinya)

Here the mundane nature of sexism is recognised as well as the responsibility of every man to make a difference. Another volunteer reflects on his own adolescence and lack of resources available then for questioning taken-for-granted assumptions about masculinity:

> *I've had to unpick so much of what I learned about women and being a man as a teenager. Sometimes I wish someone had come to my school and told me that I didn't need to be hench, super sexual, top dog, loudmouth to be a man and Boom! along comes the Great Men project.*

Here the importance of early intervention is emphasised in order to promote positive masculinities. However, the difficulty of changing ingrained attitudes is highlighted by Mike:

> *I've always tried to be a positive agent of change by challenging my friends and colleagues when they roll out the usual boring banter but it doesn't seem to always land. The GREAT Men Project offers me a chance to make a real, positive difference and start to plant the seeds of a change by talking to young men in an honest and open way.*

Another volunteer explains how becoming a father to a daughter galvanised his pro-feminist stance and prompted him to join the project:

> *I grew up with feminist ideas all around me, but it got really real when my daughter was born and everywhere I looked was sexism sexism in the tiniest everyday things. I'm a campaigner by trade and I wanted to stand up and be counted on gender equality, not just for my daughter, but for the good of people everywhere; after all, gender inequality and stereotypical masculinity is damaging for men too.* (Paul)

There is a clear consensus that questioning conventional masculinity norms is beneficial for men and society more generally. For the volunteers, supporting younger men to rethink and repurpose masculinities is a rewarding project which helps them to nurture their own identities.

Apart from gender equality projects, men are also getting involved in tackling homophobia and heterosexism. In the UK in recent years we have seen the emergence of 'straight allies' pioneered by Stonewall, an NGO dedicated to the rights of LGBT+ citizens. The straight allies programme has focused on workplaces and Stonewall has created resources and advice to enable employees and organisations to get involved. In their 2011 report, they feature quotes from interviewees across a number of organisations, for example:

> *The explicit reason why I champion lesbian, gay, bisexual and trans issues at Salford is precisely because I'm straight. And that's a very important message, because if a heterosexual person says 'I'm leading on this issue because I believe it affects everybody' then that has a real impact.* (Martin)

Not all straight allies are men of course; nor is 'masculinity' a focus for this work. However, there are other initiatives which focus on masculinity issues in tackling homophobia and heterosexism. Recently we (Lowe and Gough 2016) have been working with a young charity, Sport Allies (http://www.sportallies.org/), to understand more about how they are combatting homophobia in sport. Starting out as an attempt to provide funds for much needed equipment, a group of rowers at Warwick University decided to produce a naked calendar. Initially they did not sell many copies but over time the calendar was promoted to the gay community and became very popular, generating income for the rowing club and, subsequently, for the birth of the new charity. Several members of the club have joined the charity and have been promoting inclusivity in sport since. Here is the testimony of one rower, Tristan:

> *I became a straight ally through my involvement with the Warwick Rowers Calendar project. Initially selling only to friends and relatives, the project started gaining momentum after it attracted the attention and very positive support of the gay community. We welcomed this attention and embraced the ability to bring a certain level of joy and support to a mass audience. It felt fitting that as the gay community were supporting us, we should do our bit to support them. The supporters of the calendar were facilitating what it was that we loved and by returning the favour with our message and donations to Sport Allies, we like to think that there's now a healthy cyclical relationship between the club and our supporters. Over time our message has been heavily influenced by what we've learnt from our supporters and the experiences they've told us about playing team sports growing up. Participating in a sport as inaccessible as rowing, we can strongly relate to the idea of having a barrier to participation. The messages of thanks we've subsequently received from our supporters explaining the difference our message has made to them range from giving people the confidence to go to the gym, to joining a rowing team, or simply feeling more comfortable in themselves. It's always humbling to hear that you've given someone the confidence to try out a sport or even be open about their sexuality.* (See Lowe and Gough 2016: 50)

Here the impact of supporting the gay community is highlighted, moving beyond increased sport and exercise participation to confidence and well-being. The photographer on the calendar project and founder of Sport Allies, Angus Malcolm, emphasises the role that straight men within sport can play in supporting LGBT+ others:

> *Until I got to know the rowers, my perception of sportsmen was almost entirely negative – I saw them as a tribe united by characteristics that included arrogance, machismo and insensitivity. This was, I suppose, my response to being*

branded a 'sissy' by the sport boys at school, and it meant that for most of my life. I felt nothing but contempt for anyone involved in sport, and for sport itself. It took the rowers to show me how wrong I was. Working with these charismatic, passionate, sensitive and courageous young men over the last seven years has enabled me to see beyond the cliché of the 'jock'. I have been able to recognise the enormous benefits of participation in team sport, the depth of the bonds that are formed between team-mates, the way that they learn to work together and the support they are able to give each other as a result. This is not a culture to be dismissed – rather, I believe that participation in team sport is an opportunity for personal growth that needs to be promoted more widely, and that it is only sport's role in perpetuating patriarchal values that must change. (See Lowe and Gough 2016: 9)

As Malcolm notes, it is interesting that even in the most traditionally het-eronormative fields such as sport there is scope for changing masculinities and inclusivity (see also Anderson 2009).

IMPLICATIONS

In sum, supportive masculinities are practised within a number of dispa-rate domains, whether it is fathers caring for their children or mates shar-ing stories and humour together in the pub. Sometimes traditional notions of masculinity are invoked in seeking and providing support and advice—for example in mainstream male-targeted magazines—and at other times the environment is conducive to the expression of softer mas-culinities, such as online support forums (e.g. for infertility issues), although the influence of conventional masculinity norms may still curtail supportive words and practices here. What is clear is that the extent and nature of support offered and received by men—and the masculinities implied therein—vary by context, with individual men's practices shaped by the situation they find themselves in as well as their own personal biog-raphies. For example, online forums provide anonymity and safety but not all men who visit these sites will want to share their stories or inter-vene to support other men. And we have observed that caring and sup-port can flourish at many levels, from interpersonal encounters with friends and family members to interactions with peers online and more public demonstrations of support through interventions with young men (e.g. great men project) and campaigning work (e.g. sport allies). Perhaps it is easier to invest hope in younger generations of boys and men who may be exposed to more inclusive ideals and programmes compared to older men (cf. Anderson 2009)—although we must not discount the (potential) contributions of middle-aged and older men in promoting more caring models of masculinity (e.g. grandfathers: see Mann et al. 2016), not romanticise young masculinities when we know that boys and young men can be involved in sexual bullying and consumption of pornography (e.g. Flood 2010). Clearly, more work is required to identify barriers and facilitators to the development of supportive masculinities within different groups and communities.

REFERENCES

Anderson, E. (2009). *Inclusive masculinity: The changing nature of masculinities.* New York: Routledge.

Anderson, E. (2014). *21st century jocks: Sporting men and contemporary heterosexuality.* Basingstoke: Palgrave.

Anstiss, D., & Lyons, A. (2014). From men to the media and back again: Help-seeking in popular men's magazines. *Journal of Health Psychology, 19*(11), 1358–1370.

Applegate, J., & Kaye, L. (1993). Male elder caregivers. In C. L. Williams (Ed.), *Doing women's work: Men in nontraditional occupations.* London: Sage.

Connell, R. W. (1995). *Masculinities.* Cambridge: Polity Press.

Courtenay, W. H. (2000). Constructions of masculinity and their influence on men's well-being: A theory of gender and health. *Social Science & Medicine, 50,* 1385–1401.

Dolan, A. (2007). 'Good luck to them if they can get it': Exploring working class men's understandings and experiences of income inequality and material standards. *Sociology of Health and Illness, 29*(5), 1–19.

Doucet, A. (2006). *Do men mother? Fatherhood, care, and domestic responsibility.* Toronto: University of Toronto Press.

Emslie, C., Hunt, K., & Lyons, A. (2013). The role of alcohol in forging and maintaining friendships amongst Scottish men in midlife. *Health Psychology, 32*(1), 33–41.

Finn, M., & Henwood, K. L. (2009). Exploring masculinities within men's identificatory imaginings of first time fatherhood. *British Journal of Social Psychology, 48*(3), 547–562.

Flood, M. (2010). Young men using porn. In K. Boyle (Ed.), *Everyday pornographies.* London: Routledge.

Fraser, C., & Warr, D. J. (2009). Challenging roles: Insights into issues for men caring for family members with mental illness. *American Journal of Men's Health, 3*(1), 36–49.

Gough, B. (2016). Men's depression talk online: A qualitative analysis of accountability and authenticity in help-seeking and support formulations. *Psychology of Men & Masculinity, 17,* 156–165.

Gough, B., & Edwards, G. (1998). The beer talking: Four lads, a carry out and the reproduction of masculinities. *The Sociological Review, 46*(3), 409–455.

Hall, M., Gough, B., & Seymour-Smith, S. (2012a). 'I'm METRO, NOT gay', a discursive analysis of men's make-up use on YouTube. *Journal of Men's Studies, 20*(3), 209–226.

Hall, M., Gough, B., & Seymour-Smith, S. (2012b). On-line constructions of metrosexuality and masculinities: A membership categorisation analysis. *Gender and Language, 6*(2), 379–403.

Hall, M., Grogan, S., & Gough, B. (2015). 'It is safe to use if you are healthy': A discursive analysis of men's online accounts of ephedrine use. *Psychology & Health, 30*(7), 770–782.

Hanlon, N. (2012). *Masculinities, care and equality: Identity and nurture in men's lives.* Basingstoke: Palgrave.

Hanna, E., & Gough, B. (2016). Searching for help online: An analysis of peer-to-peer posts on a male-only infertility forum. *Journal of Health Psychology,* 1–12. https://doi.org/10.1177/1359105316644038.

Hunter, C., Riggs, D. W., & Augoustinos, M. (2017). Constructions of primary caregiving fathers in popular parenting texts. *Men and Masculinities.* https://doi.org/10.1177/1097184X17730593.

Lomas, T. (2013). Critical positive masculinity. *MSC-Masculinities & Social Change, 2*(2), 167–193.

Lowe, A., & Gough, B. (2016). *Homophobia, gender and sporting culture.* London: Sport Allies.

Lynch, K., Baker, J., Walsh, J., & Lyons, M. (Eds.). (2009). *Affective equality: Who cares? Love, care and injustice.* London: Palgrave Macmillan.

Mann, R., Tarrant, A., & Leeson, G. (2016). Grandfatherhood: Shifting masculinities in later life. *Sociology, 50*(3), 594–610.

McQueen, F. (2017). Male emotionality: 'Boys don't cry' versus 'it's good to talk'. *NORMA: International Journal for Masculinity Studies, 12*(3–4). https://doi.org/10.1080/18902138.2017.1336877.

O'Neill, R. (2015). Whither critical masculinity studies? Notes on inclusive masculinity theory, Postfeminism, and sexual politics. *Men and Masculinities, 18*(1), 100–120.

ONS. (2016). *Women shoulder the responsibility of unpaid work.* London: Office for National Statistics.

Peralta, R. L. (2007). College alcohol use and the embodiment of hegemonic masculinity among European American men. *Sex Roles, 56*(11/12), 741–756.

Ricciardelli, R., Clow, K., & White, P. (2010). Investigating hegemonic masculinity: Portrayals of masculinity in men's lifestyle magazines. *Sex Roles, 63,* 64–78.

Robertson, S. (2007). *Understanding men and health: Masculinities, identity and well-being.* Buckingham: Open University Press.

Robinson, V., Hall, A., & Hockey, J. (2011). Masculinities, sexualities, and the limits of subversion: Being a man in hairdressing. *Men and Masculinities, 14*(1), 31–50.

Rochlen, A. B., Paterniti, D. A., Epstein, R. M., Duberstein, P., Willeford, L., & Kravitz, R. L. (2010). Barriers in diagnosing and treating men with depression: A focus group report. *American Journal of Men's Health, 4,* 167–175.

Scambor, E., Bergmann, N., Wojnicka, K., Belghiti-Mahut, S., Hearn, J., Holter, O. G., Gärtner, M., Hrženjak, M., Scambor, C., & White, A. (2014). Men and gender equality: European insights. *Men & Masculinities, 17,* 552–577.

Stevenson, N., Jackson, P., & Brooks, K. (2000). The politics of 'new' men's lifestyle magazines. *European Journal of Cultural Studies, 3,* 366–385.

Stibbe, A. (2004). Health and the social construction of masculinity in Men's health magazine. *Men & Masculinities, 7,* 31–51.

Weinland, J. A. (2009). The lived experience of informal African American male caregivers. *American Journal of Men's Health, 3*(1), 16–24.

AFTERWORD

This short book has presented an analysis of contemporary masculinities as evolving, convoluted, and rich, with men grappling with conventional and modern ideals and practices relating to their bodies, emotions, and relationship with self and others. It perhaps chimes with increasingly sophisticated depictions (and deconstructions) of men and masculinity within popular culture. In the popular US sitcom *Modern Family*, for example, even Jay, the grizzled patriarch, is shown to have 'soft' moments while Phil, the ostensibly more evolved and gentle son-in-law, is sometimes seen to seek more traditional masculine approval (the rendering of gay masculinity in the characters of the married couple Cam and Mitch is similarly nuanced). In the UK, a recent bestselling autobiography by the comic actor and writer Robert Webb portrays the struggles with and pointlessness of traditional masculinity norms (title: 'How not to be a boy'). Of course, these characterisations sit alongside more one-dimensional and normative constructions of masculinity within popular culture, but arguably we are now witnessing an expansion in the repertoires of masculinity available.

Broadly, I paint a (critically) positive portrait in the book, drawing attention to progress and possibilities, with (some) men now caring more for their own well-being and that of others and in so doing rejecting or reworking traditional gender scripts. At the same time, this (cautiously) optimistic tone must be informed by continuing constraints and contradictions; for example, while more men are learning to articulate their

© The Author(s) 2018   75
B. Gough, *Contemporary Masculinities*,
https://doi.org/10.1007/978-3-319-78819-7

feelings and needs, at least in certain 'safe' contexts (e.g. online forums), the statistics for male suicide remain worryingly high, suggesting that a significant number of men and boys struggle with emotional expression and help-seeking. Although several interventions have been designed to tackle this issue in several countries, more resources and initiatives are required within mental health promotion to reach more men.

An important point emphasised in the book is the need to consider how masculinities are intersected by other pertinent social identity categories such as race, sexual orientation, and social class. Increasingly, masculinity scholars are exploring how masculinity is constructed and constrained in relation to particular communities of men; for example, considering how black and minority ethnic men negotiate masculinity in the context of racism or how white working-class men experience assimilation into neoliberal gig economy working arrangements. Age is another interesting dimension—how are different generations responding to contemporary images of masculinity, and how is masculinity enacted within diverse environments (school, workplace, family)?

Finally, the rising number of boys and men involved in campaigns for gender equality is a heartening phenomenon. Across the world there is evidence of male engagement in a range of programmes designed to challenge 'toxic' iterations of masculinity and to promote the welfare and status of girls and women and marginalised groups of men. More generally, there seems to be more media and public awareness of problems associated with men and masculinity, as evidenced by the outcry and campaigning post-Weinstein (cf. #metoo), and a genuine appetite to tackle sexism, sexual exploitation, and inequalities. Although the current political climate also promotes conservative and men's rights agendas in several Western societies, this does not detract from the parallel efforts to promote a fairer society which values more tolerant, inclusive masculinities and equality between men and women.

REFERENCES

Adams, G., Turner, H., & Bucks, R. (2005). The experience of body dissatisfaction in men. *Body Image, 2*(3), 271–283.

Addis, M. E. (2008). Gender and depression in men. *Clinical Psychology: Science and Practice, 15,* 153–168.

Addis, M. E., & Mahalik, J. (2003). Men, masculinity and the contexts of help seeking. *American Psychologist, 58*(1), 5–14.

Advisory Council on the Misuse of Drugs. (2010). *Consideration of the anabolic steroids.* UK Government. Retrieved from https://www.gov.uk/government/publications/advisory-council-on-the-misuse-of-drugs-consideration-of-the-anabolic-steroids—2

Aitkenhead, D. (2005, September 14). Most British woman now expect to have cosmetic surgery in their lifetime: How did the ultimate feminist taboo become just another lifestyle choice? *The Guardian,* p. 13.

Anderson, E. (2005). Orthodox and inclusive masculinity: Competing masculinities among heterosexual men in a feminized terrain. *Sociological Perspectives, 48,* 337–355.

Anderson, E. (2008). Being masculine is not about who you sleep with...:' Heterosexual athletes contesting masculinity and the one-time rule of homosexuality. *Sex Roles, 58*(1–2), 104–115.

Anderson, E. (2009). *Inclusive masculinity: The changing nature of masculinities.* New York: Routledge.

Anderson, E. (2014). *21st century jocks: Sporting men and contemporary heterosexuality.* Basingstoke: Palgrave.

Andrews, M., Day Sclater, S., Squire, C., & Tamboukou, M. (2004). Narrative research. In C. Seale, D. Silverman, J. Gubrium, & G. Gobo (Eds.), *Qualitative research practice* (pp. 97–112). London: Sage.

Anstiss, D., & Lyons, A. (2014). From men to the media and back again: Help-seeking in popular men's magazines. *Journal of Health Psychology, 19*(11), 1358–1370.

© The Author(s) 2018
B. Gough, *Contemporary Masculinities,*
https://doi.org/10.1007/978-3-319-78819-7

Applegate, J., & Kaye, L. (1993). Male elder caregivers. In C. L. Williams (Ed.), *Doing women's work: Men in nontraditional occupations.* London: Sage.

Atkinson, M. (2010). *Deconstructing men and masculinities.* Toronto: Oxford University Press.

Banks, I. (2005). *The HGV man manual.* Somerset: Haynes Publishing.

Barnes, L. (2014). *Conceiving masculinity: Male infertility, medicine, and identity.* Philadelphia: Temple University Press.

Bem, S. L. (1974). The measurement of psychological androgyny. *Journal of Consulting and Clinical Psychology, 42,* 155–162.

Bennett, E., & Gough, B. (2013). In pursuit of leanness: Constructing bodies and masculinities online within a men's weight management forum. *Health, 17*(3), 284–299.

Bordo, S. (1993). *Unbearable weight: Feminism, western culture and the body.* Berkeley: University of California Press.

Bordo, S. (1999). *The male body: A new look at men in public and in private* (1st paperback ed.). New York: Farrar, Straus & Giroux Inc.

Bourdieu, P. (1986). The forms of capital. In I. Szeman & T. Kaposy, (Eds.). (2011) *Cultural theory: An anthology* (pp. 81–93). Chichester: John Wiley & Sons, Ltd.

Brannon, D. (1976). The male sex role: Our culture's blueprint for manhood and what it's done for us lately. In D. Brannon (Ed.), *The forty-nine percent majority: The male sex role.* Reading: Addison-Wesley.

Braun, V., Clarke, V., & Gray, D. (Eds.). (2017). *Collecting qualitative data: A practical guide to textual, media and virtual methods.* Cambridge: Cambridge University Press.

Bridges, T., & Pascoe, C. J. (2014). Hybrid masculinities: New directions in the sociology of men and masculinities. *Sociology Compass, 8*(3), 246–258.

Broom, A., & Tovey, P. (Eds.). (2009). *Men's health: Body, identity and social context.* Oxford: Wiley-Blackwell.

Brown, T. A., & Keel, P. K. (2015). A randomized controlled trial of a peer co-led dissonance-based eating disorder prevention program for gay men. *Behaviour Research and Therapy, 74,* 1–10.

Brownhill, S., Wilhelm, K., Barclay, L., & Schmied, V. (2005). 'Big Build': hidden depression in men. *Australian and New Zealand Journal of Psychiatry, 39*(10), 921–931.

Burkitt, I. (2002). Complex emotions: Relations, feelings and images in emotional experience. *The Sociological Review, 50*(S2), 151–167.

Bye, C., Avery, A., & Lavin, J. (2005). Tackling obesity in men - preliminary evaluation of men only groups within a commercial slimming organization. *Journal of Human Nutrition and Dietetics, 18,* 391–394.

Calasanti, T., Pietila, I., Ojala, H., & King, N. (2013). Men, bodily control, and health behaviours: The importance of age. *Health Psychology, 32*(1), 15–23.

Calfee, R., & Fadale, F. (2006). Popular ergogenic drugs and supplements in young athletes. *Pediatrics, 117*, 577–589.

Carrigan, T., Connell, R. W., & Lee, J. (1985). Toward a new sociology of masculinity. *Theory and Society, 14*, 551–604.

Childs, D. (2007). Like implants for the arms: Synthol lures bodybuilders. *ABC News*. Available at: http://abcnews.go.com/Health/Fitness/story?id=3179969

Clare, A. (2000). *On men: Masculinity in crisis*. London: Chatto and Windus.

Cleland, J. (2013). Book review: Inclusive masculinity: The changing nature of masculinities. *International Review for the Sociology of Sport, 48*(3), 380–383.

Coad, D. (2008). *The metrosexual: Gender, sexuality, and sport*. New York: State University of New York Press.

Cole, E. R. (2009). Intersectionality and research in psychology. *American Psychologist, 64*, 170–180.

Collier, R. (1992). The new man: fact or fad? *Achilles Heel*. Retrieved June 6, 2009, from http://www.achillesheel.freeuk.com/article14_9.html

Connell, R. W. (1995). *Masculinities*. Cambridge: Polity Press.

Connell, R. W. (2005). *Masculinities* (2nd ed.). Cambridge: Polity Press.

Connell, R. W., & Messerschmidt, J. W. (2005). Hegemonic masculinity rethinking the concept. *Gender & Society, 19*(6), 829–859.

Courtenay, W. H. (2000). Constructions of masculinity and their influence on men's well-being: A theory of gender and health. *Social Science & Medicine, 50*, 1385–1401.

Crawford, R. (2006). Health as a meaningful social practice. *Health, 10*(4), 401–420.

Crawshaw, P. (2007). Governing the healthy male citizen: Men, masculinity, and popular health in Men's Health magazine. *Social Science & Medicine, 65*, 1606–1618.

Cudmore, L. (2005). Becoming parents in the context of loss. *Sexual and Relationship Therapy, 20*, 299–308.

Culley, L., Hudson, N., & Hohan, M. (2013). Where are all the men? The marginalization of men in social scientific research on infertility. *Reproductive Biomedicine Online, 27*, 225–235.

Davidson, K., & Meadows, R. (2010). Older men's health: The role of marital status and masculinities. In B. Gough & S. Robertson (Eds.), *Men, masculinities & health: Critical* (pp. 109–124). Basingstoke: Palgrave.

De Boise, S., & Hearn, J. (2017). Are men getting more emotional? Critical sociological perspectives on men, masculinities and emotion. *The Sociological Review*, 1–18.

de Visser, R. O., & McDonnell, E. J. (2013). 'Man points': Masculine capital and young men's health. *Health Psychology, 32*(1), 5–14.

de Visser, R. O., Smith, J. A., & McDonnell, E. J. (2009). 'That's not masculine': Masculine capital and health-related behaviour. *Journal of Health Psychology, 14*(7), 1047–1058.

Demetriou, D. Z. (2001). Connell's concept of hegemonic masculinity: A critique. *Theory & Society, 30*(3), 337–361.

Dolan, A. (2007). 'Good luck to them if they can get it': Exploring working class men's understandings and experiences of income inequality and material standards. *Sociology of Health and Illness, 29*(5), 1–19.

Doucet, A. (2006). *Do men mother? Fatherhood, care, and domestic responsibility.* Toronto: University of Toronto Press.

Drummond, M. J. (2011). Reflections on the archetypal heterosexual male body. *Australian Feminist Studies, 26*(67), 103–117.

Drummond, M., & Gough, B. (in press). Men, body image and cancer. In M. Fingeret & I. Teo (Eds.), *Principles and practices of body image care for cancer patients.*

Edwards, C., Tod, D., & Molnar, G. (2014). A systematic review of the drive for muscularity research area. *International Review of Sport and Exercise Psychology, 7,* 18–41.

Elliott, K. (2016). Caring masculinities: Theorising an emerging concept. *Men & Masculinities, 19*(3), 240–259.

Emslie, C., Hunt, K., & Lyons, A. (2013). The role of alcohol in forging and maintaining friendships amongst Scottish men in midlife. *Health Psychology, 32*(1), 33–41.

Featherstone, M. (1991). The body in consumer culture. In M. Featherstone, M. Hepworth, & B. S. Turner (Eds.), *The body: Social process and cultural theory* (pp. 170–196). London: Sage.

Filiault, S. M., Drummond, M. J., & Smith, J. (2008). Gay men and prostate cancer: Voicing the concerns of a hidden population. *Journal of Men's Health, 5*(4), 327–332.

Finn, M., & Henwood, K. L. (2009). Exploring masculinities within men's identificatory imaginings of first time fatherhood. *British Journal of Social Psychology, 48*(3), 547–562.

Flood, M. (2010). Young men using porn. In K. Boyle (Ed.), *Everyday pornographies.* London: Routledge.

For Him Magazine (FHM). (2009–10). Advice columns and letter/reply sections. (November 2009–February 2010).

Fraser, C., & Warr, D. J. (2009). Challenging roles: Insights into issues for men caring for family members with mental illness. *American Journal of Men's Health, 3*(1), 36–49.

Galasinski, D. (2008). *Men's discourses of depression.* Basingstoke: Palgrave.

Giddens, A. (1991). *Modernity and self-identity: Self and society in the late modern age.* Cambridge: Polity Press.

Gill, R., Henwood, K., & McLean, C. (2005). Body projects and the regulation of normative masculinity. *Body and Society, 11*(1), 39–62.

Gough, B. (2007). 'Real men don't diet': An analysis of contemporary newspaper representations of men, food and health. *Social Science & Medicine, 64*(2), 326–337.

Gough, B. (2009). Promoting 'masculinity' over health: A critical analysis of Men's health promotion with particular reference to an obesity reduction 'manual'. In B. Gough & S. Robertson (Eds.), *Men, masculinities and health: Critical perspectives.* Basingstoke: Palgrave.

Gough, B. (2013). The psychology of men's health: Maximizing masculine capital. *Health Psychology, 32*(1), 1–4.

Gough, B. (2016). Men's depression talk online: A qualitative analysis of accountability and authenticity in help-seeking and support formulations. *Psychology of Men & Masculinity, 17,* 156–165.

Gough, B., & Edwards, G. (1998). The beer talking: Four lads, a carry out and the reproduction of masculinities. *The Sociological Review, 46*(3), 409–455.

Gough, B., & Flanders, G. (2009). Celebrating 'Obese' bodies: Gay 'Bears' talk about weight, body image and health. *International Journal of Men's Health, 8*(3), 235–253.

Gough, B., & Lyons, A. (2016). The future of qualitative research in psychology: Accentuating the positive. *IPBS: Integrative Psychological & Behavioral Science, 50*(2), 243–252.

Gough, B., & Madill, A. (2012). Subjectivity in psychological science: From problem to prospect. *Psychological Methods, 17*(3), 374–384.

Gough, B., & Robertson, S. (Eds.). (2009). *Men, masculinities and health: Critical perspectives.* Basingstoke: Palgrave.

Gough, B., Hall, M., & Seymour-Smith, S. (2014). Straight guys do wear make-up: Contemporary masculinities and investment in appearance. In S. Roberts (Ed.), *Debating modern masculinities: Change, continuity, crisis?* (pp. 106–124). Basingstoke: Palgrave Macmillan.

Gough, B., Seymour-Smith, S., & Matthews, C. R. (2016). Body dissatisfaction, appearance investment and wellbeing: How older obese men orient to 'aesthetic health'. *Psychology of Men & Masculinity, 17*(1), 84–91.

Gray, J. J., & Ginsberg, R. L. (2007). Muscle dissatisfaction: An overview of psychological and cultural research and theory. In J. K. Thompson & G. Cafri (Eds.), *The muscular ideal: Psychological, social, and medical perspectives* (pp. 15–39). Washington, DC: American Psychological Association.

Gray, C., Anderson, A., Dalziel, A., Hunt, K., Leishman, J., & Wyke, S. (2009). Addressing male obesity: An evaluation of a group-based weight management intervention for Scottish men. *Journal of Men's Health and Gender, 6,* 70–81.

Green, G., Emslie, C., O'Neill, D., Hunt, K., & Walker, S. (2010). Exploring the ambiguities of masculinity in accounts of emotional distress in the military among ex-servicemen. *Social Science & Medicine, 71*(8), 1480–1488.

Griffith, D., Allen, J. O., & Gunter, K. (2011). Social and cultural factors influence African American men's medical help seeking. *Research on Social Work Practice, 21*, 337–347.

Grogan, S. (2008). *Body image: Understanding body dissatisfaction in men, women, and children*. London: Routledge.

Gross, J. (2005). Phat. In D. Kulick & A. Meneley (Eds.), *Fat: The anthropology of an obsession* (pp. 63–76). New York: Penguin.

Hale, S., Grogan, S., & Willott, S. (2010). Male GPs' views on men seeking medical help: A qualitative study. *British Journal of Health Psychology, 15*(4), 697–713.

Hall, M. (2015). 'When there's no underbrush the tree looks taller': A discourse analysis of men's online groin shaving talk. *Sexualities, 18*(8), 997–1017.

Hall, M., Gough, B., & Hansen, S. (2011). Magazine and reader constructions of 'metrosexuality' and masculinity: A membership categorisation analysis. *Journal of Gender Studies, 20*(1), 69–87.

Hall, M., Gough, B., & Seymour-Smith, S. (2012a). 'I'm METRO, NOT gay', a discursive analysis of men's make-up use on YouTube. *Journal of Men's Studies, 20*(3), 209–226.

Hall, M., Gough, B., & Seymour-Smith, S. (2012b). On-line constructions of metrosexuality and masculinities: A membership categorisation analysis. *Gender and Language, 6*(2), 379–403.

Hall, M., Grogan, S., & Gough, B. (2015). 'It is safe to use if you are healthy': A discursive analysis of men's online accounts of ephedrine use. *Psychology & Health, 30*(7), 770–782.

Hamilton, C. J., & Mahalik, J. R. (2009). Minority stress, masculinity, and social norms predicting gay men's health risk behaviors. *Journal of Counseling Psychology, 56*, 132–141.

Hanlon, N. (2012). *Masculinities, care and equality: Identity and nurture in men's lives*. Basingstoke: Palgrave.

Hanna, E., & Gough, B. (2016a). Emoting infertility online: A qualitative analysis of men's forum posts. *Health, 20*(4), 363–382.

Hanna, E., & Gough, B. (2016b). Searching for help online: An analysis of peer-to-peer posts on a male-only infertility forum. *Journal of Health Psychology*, 1–12. https://doi.org/10.1177/1359105316644038.

Hearn, J. (1996). Is masculinity dead?: A critique of the concept masculinity/masculinities. In M. Mac an Ghaill (Ed.), *Understanding masculinities* (pp. 202–217). Buckingham: Open University Press.

Hearn, J. (2004). From hegemonic masculinity to the hegemony of men. *Feminist Theory, 5*(1), 49–72.

Hunt, K., Wyke, S., Gray, C. M., Anderson, A. S., Brady, A., Bunn, C., Donnan, P. T., Fenwick, E., Grieve, E., Leishman, J., Miller, E., Mutrie, N., Rauchhaus, P., White, A., & Treweek, S. (2014). A gender-sensitised weight loss and healthy living programme for overweight and obese men delivered by Scottish premier league football clubs (FFIT): A pragmatic randomised controlled trial. *The Lancet, 383*, 1211–1221.

Hunter, C., Riggs, D. W., & Augoustinos, M. (2017). Constructions of primary caregiving fathers in popular parenting texts. *Men and Masculinities.* https://doi.org/10.1177/1097184X17730593.

Immergut, M. (2010). Manscaping: The tangle of nature, culture and male body hair. In L. Moore & M. E. Kosut (Eds.), *The body reader: Essential social and cultural readings* (pp. 287–304). New York: New York University Press.

Ingram, N., & Waller, R. (2014). Degrees of masculinity: Working and middle class undergraduate students' constructions of masculine identities. In S. Roberts (Ed.), *Debating modern masculinities.* London: Palgrave Macmillan.

Iwamoto, D. K., Cheng, A., Lee, C. S., Takamatsu, S., & Gordon, D. (2011). 'Man-ing' up and getting drunk: The role of masculine norms, alcohol intoxication and alcohol-related problems among college men. *Addictive Behavior, 36*(9), 906–911.

Jankowski, G. S., Fawkner, H., Slater, A., & Tiggemann, M. (2014). 'Appearance potent'? Are gay men's magazines more "appearance potent" than straight men's magazines in the UK? *Body Image, 11*(4), 474–481.

Jankowski, G., Gough, B., Fawkner, H., Diedrichs, P.C., & Halliwell, E. (submitted). It affects me, it affects me not: The impact of men's body dissatisfaction.

Johnson, J. L., Oliffe, J. L., Kelly, M. T., Galdas, P., & Ogrodniczuk, J. S. (2012). Men's discourses of help-seeking in the context of depression. *Sociology of Health & Illness, 34*, 345–361.

Kahn, J. (2009). *An introduction to masculinities.* Oxford: Wiley Blackwell.

Kanayama, G., Barry, S., Hudson, J. I., & Pope, H. G., Jr. (2006). Body image and attitudes toward male roles in anabolic-androgenic steroid users. *American Journal of Psychiatry, 163*(4), 697–703.

Karepova, M. (2010). *Psychological counselling in Russia: The making of a feminised profession.* PhD Thesis, University of York, UK.

Kehler, M., & Atkinson, M. (Eds.). (2010). *Boys' bodies: Speaking the unspoken.* New York: Peter Lang.

Kim, B. S., Atkinson, D. R., & Umemoto, D. (2001). Asian cultural values and the counseling process: Current knowledge and directions for future research. *The Counseling Psychologist, 29*(4), 570–603.

Kimmel, M. (2013). *Angry white men: American masculinity at the end of an era.* New York: Nation Books/Perseus.

Kozinets, R. V. (2002). The field behind the screen: Using the method of netnography to research market-oriented virtual communities. *Journal of Consumer Research, 39*(1), 61–72.

Labre, M. P. (2005). Burn fat, build muscle: A content analysis of men's health and men's fitness. *International Journal of Men's Health, 4*(2), 187–200.

Lazarus, R. S., & Folkman, S. (1984). *Stress, appraisal and coping*. New York: Springer.

Levant, R. F. (2011). Research in the psychology of men and masculinity using the gender role strain paradigm as a framework. *American Psychologist, 66*(8), 765–776.

Levant, R. F., Rankin, T. J., Williams, C., Hasan, N. T., & Smalley, K. B. (2010). Evaluation of the factor structure and construct validity of the male role norms inventory-revised (MRNI-R). *Psychology of Men & Masculinity, 11*, 25–37.

Levant, R. F., Wimer, D. J., & Williams, C. M. (2011). An evaluation of the psychometric properties of the health behavior Inventory-20 (HBI-20) and its relationships to masculinity and attitudes towards seeking psychological help among college men. *Psychology of Men and Masculinity, 11*, 26–41.

Liossi, C. (2003). *Appearance related concerns across the general and clinical populations*. London: City University. Retrieved from http://ukpmc.ac.uk/theses/ETH/407535

Lomas, T. (2013). Critical positive masculinity. *MSC-Masculinities & Social Change, 2*(2), 167–193.

Lomas, T. (2014). *Masculinity, meditation, and mental health*. Basingstoke: Palgrave.

Lomas, T., Cartwright, T., Edginton, T., & Ridge, D. (2016). New ways of being a man: Positive hegemonic masculinity in meditation-based communities of practice. *Men and Masculinities, 19*, 289–310.

Lowe, A., & Gough, B. (2016). *Homophobia, gender and sporting culture*. London: Sport Allies.

Lupton, B. (2000). Maintaining masculinity: Men who do women's work. *British Journal of Management, 11*(S1), 33–48.

Lynch, K., Baker, J., Walsh, J., & Lyons, M. (Eds.). (2009). *Affective equality: Who cares? Love, care and injustice*. London: Palgrave Macmillan.

Mac an Ghaill, M., & Haywood, C. (2012). Understanding boys: Thinking through boys, masculinity and suicide. *Social Science and Medicine, 74*(4), 482–489.

MacDonald, J. (2011). Building on the strength of Australian males. *International Journal of Men's Health, 10*, 82–96.

Mahalik, J. R., Locke, B., Ludlow, L., Diemer, M., Scott, R. P. J., Gottfried, M., & Freitas, G. (2003). Development of the conformity to masculine norms inventory. *Psychology of Men and Masculinity, 4*, 3–25.

Malik, A., & Coulson, N. (2008). The male experience of infertility: A thematic analysis of an online infertility support group bulletin board. *Journal of Reproductive and Infant Psychology, 26*, 18–30.

Mann, R., Tarrant, A., & Leeson, G. (2016). Grandfatherhood: Shifting masculinities in later life. *Sociology, 50*(3), 594–610.

McCormack, M. (2011). Hierarchy without hegemony: Locating boys in an inclusive school setting. *Sociological Perspectives, 54*(1), 83–101.

McCormack, M. (2012). *The declining significance of homophobia: How teenage boys are redefining masculinity and heterosexuality.* Oxford/New York: Oxford University Press.

McCormack, M., & Anderson, E. (2010). It's just not acceptable any more: The erosion of homophobia and the softening of masculinity at an English sixth form. *Sociology, 44*(5), 843–859.

McCreary, D. R., & Sasse, D. K. (2000). An exploration of the drive for muscularity in adolescent boys and girls. *Journal of American College Health, 48,* 297–304.

McQueen, F. (2017). Male emotionality: 'Boys don't cry' versus 'it's good to talk'. *NORMA: International Journal for Masculinity Studies, 12*(3–4). https://doi.org/10.1080/18902138.2017.1336877.

Mellor, D., Fuller-Tyszkiewicz, M., McCabe, M. P., & Ricciardelli, L. A. (2010). Body image and self-esteem across age and gender: A short-term longitudinal study. *Sex Roles, 63*(9–10), 672–681.

Men's Health Magazine. (2009–10) Advice columns and letter/reply sections. (November 2009–February 2010).

Miller, T. (2005). A metrosexual eye on queer guy. *GLQ: A Journal of Lesbian and Gay Studies, 11,* 112–117.

Miller, T. (2009). *Metrosexuality: See the bright light of commodification shine! Watch yanqui masculinity made over.* Paper presented at the annual meeting of the American Studies Association, 24 May, Accessed 12 May 2010 from http://www.allacademic.com/meta/p105600_index. html

Monaghan, L. F. (2005). Big handsome men, bears and others: Virtual constructions of 'fat male embodiment'. *Body & Society, 11*(2), 81–111.

Monaghan, L. F. (2007). Body mass index, masculinities and moral worth: Men's critical understandings of 'appropriate' weight-for-health. *Sociology of Health & Illness, 29*(4), 584–609.

Monaghan, L. F. (2008). Men, physical activity and the obesity discourse: Critical understandings from a qualitative study. *Sociology of Sport Journal: Special Issue on the Social Construction of Fat, 25*(1), 97–128.

Moore, S. (1989). Getting a bit of the other – The pimps of postmodernism. In R. Chapman & J. Rutherford (Eds.), *Male order: Unwrapping masculinity* (pp. 165–192). London: Lawrence & Wishart.

Morison, L., Trigeorgis, C., & John, M. (2014). Are mental health services inherently feminised? *The Psychologist, 27,* 414–417.

Morris, M., & Anderson, E. (2015). 'Charlie is so cool like': Authenticity, popularity and inclusive masculinity on YouTube. *Sociology, 49*(6), 1200–1217.

Murray, S., Rieger, E., Touyz, S. W., & De La Garcia, Y. (2010). Muscle dysmorphia and the DSM-V conundrum: Where does it belong? A review paper. *International Journal of Eating Disorders, 43*(6), 483–491.

Noone, J. H., & Stephens, C. (2008). Men, masculine idendities, and health care utilisation. *Sociology of Health & Illness, 30*(5), 711–725.

O'Neil, J. M. (1981). Patterns of gender role conflict and strain: Sexism and fear of femininity in men's lives. *Personnel and Guidance Journal, 60,* 203–210.

O'Neil, J. M., Helm, B., Gable, R., David, L., & Wrightsman, L. (1986). Gender role conflict scale (GRCS): College men's fears of femininity. *Sex Roles, 14,* 335–350.

O'Neill, J. (2008). Summarizing 25 years of research on men's gender role conflict using the gender role conflict scale: New research paradigms and clinical implications. *The Counseling Psychologist, 36,* 358–445.

O'Neill, R. (2015). Whither critical masculinity studies? Notes on inclusive masculinity theory, Postfeminism, and sexual politics. *Men and Masculinities, 18*(1), 100–120.

Oakley, L. (2011). *The epidemiology of infertility: Measurement, prevalence and an investigation of early life and reproductive, risk factors.* PhD Thesis, London School of Hygiene and Tropical Medicine. Available at: http://researchonline.lshtm.ac.uk/682432/1/549753.pdf. Accessed 17 Sept 2015.

Oliffe, J. L., Han, C. S., Ogrodniczuk, J. S., Phillips, J. C., & Roy, P. (2011). Suicide from the perspectives of older men who experience depression: A gender analysis. *American Journal of Men's Health, 5,* 444–454.

Oliffe, J., Ogrodniczuk, J. S., Bottorff, J. L., Johnson, J. L., & Hoyak, K. (2012). 'You feel like you can't live anymore': Suicide from the perspectives of Canadian men who experience depression. *Social Science & Medicine, 74*(4), 506–514.

Olivardia, R., Pope, H. G., Jr., Borowiecki, J. J., & Cohane, G. H. (2004). Biceps and body image: The relationship between muscularity and self-esteem, depression, and eating disorder symptoms. *Psychology of Men & Masculinity, 5*(2), 112–120.

ONS. (2016). *Women shoulder the responsibility of unpaid work.* London: Office for National Statistics.

ONS. (2017). *Suicides in the UK: 2016 registrations.* London: Office for National Statistics.

Paechter, C. (2003). Masculinities and feminities as communities of practice. *Women's Studies International Forum, 26*(1), 69–77.

Parrott, D. J. (2009). Aggression toward gay men as gender role enforcement: Effects of male role norms, sexual prejudice, and masculine gender role stress. *Journal of Personality, 77,* 1137–1166.

Pease, B. (2012). The politics of gendered emotions: Disrupting men's emotional investment in privilege. *Australian Journal of Social Issues, 47,* 125–142.

Peralta, R. L. (2007). College alcohol use and the embodiment of hegemonic masculinity among European American men. *Sex Roles, 56*(11/12), 741–756.

Phoenix, C., & Sparkes, A. C. (2009). Being Fred: Big stories, small stories and the accomplishment of a positive ageing identity. *Qualitative Research, 9*(2), 219–236.

Pleck, J. (1981). *The myth of masculinity.* Cambridge, MA: MIT Press.

Pope, H. G., Jr., Phillips, K. A., & Olivardia, R. (2000). *The Adonis Complex: The secret crisis of male body obsession*. New York: Free Press.

Potter, J., & Hepburn, A. (2005). Qualitative interviews in psychology: Problems and possibilities. *Qualitative Research in Psychology, 2*(4), 281–307.

Pronger, B. (1999). Outta my endzone: Sport and the territorial anus. *Journal of Sport and Social Issues, 23*, 373–389.

Pullen, A., & Simpson, R. (2009). Managing difference in feminized work: Men, otherness and social practice. *Human Relations, 62*(4), 561–587.

Ricciardelli, L. A. (2012). Body image development- adolescent boys. In T. Cash (Ed.), *Encyclopedia of body image and human appearance* (pp. 180–187). London: Elsevier.

Ricciardelli, L. A., McCabe, M. P., & Ridge, D. (2006). The construction of the adolescent male body through sport. *Journal of Health Psychology, 11*, 577–587.

Ricciardelli, R., Clow, K., & White, P. (2010). Investigating hegemonic masculinity: Portrayals of masculinity in men's lifestyle magazines. *Sex Roles, 63*, 64–78.

Richards, D. A., & Borglin, G. (2011). Implementation of psychological therapies for anxiety and depression in routine practice: Two year prospective cohort study. *Journal of Affective Disorders, 133*, 51–60.

Ricoeur, P. (1970). *Freud and philosophy: An essay on interpretation* (D. Savage, Trans.). New Haven: Yale University Press.

Riessman, C. K. (2008). *Narrative methods for the human sciences*. London: Sage.

Robertson, S. (2006). I've been like a coiled spring this last week': Embodied masculinity and health. *Sociology of Health and Illness, 28*(4), 433–456.

Robertson, S. (2007). *Understanding men and health: Masculinities, identity and well-being*. Buckingham: Open University Press.

Robertson, S., & Monaghan, L. (2012). Embodied heterosexual masculinities part 2: Foregrounding Men's health and emotions. *Sociology Compass, 6*(2), 151–165.

Robertson, S., Sheik, K., & Moore, A. (2010). Embodied masculinities in the context of cardiac rehabilitation. *Sociology of Health & Illness, 32*(5), 695–710.

Robertson, S., Witty, K., Zwolinsky, S., & Day, R. (2013). Men's health promotion interventions: What have we learned from previous programmes? *Community Practitioner, 86*(11), 38–41.

Robertson, S., Williams, B., & Oliffe, J. (2016). The case for retaining a focus on "masculinities" in Men's Health Research. *International Journal of Men's Health, 15*(1), 52–67.

Robertson, S., Gough, B., & Robinson, M. (2017). Masculinities and health inequalities within neoliberal economies. In C. Walker & S. Roberts (Eds.), *Masculinity, labour, and neoliberalism: Working-class men in international perspective*. Basingstoke: Palgrave Macmillan.

Robinson, V., Hall, A., & Hockey, J. (2011). Masculinities, sexualities, and the limits of subversion: Being a man in hairdressing. *Men and Masculinities, 14*(1), 31–50.

Rochlen, A. B., Paterniti, D. A., Epstein, R. M., Duberstein, P., Willeford, L., & Kravitz, R. L. (2010). Barriers in diagnosing and treating men with depression: A focus group report. *American Journal of Men's Health, 4*, 167–175.

Rothgerber, H. (2012). Real men don't eat (vegetable) quiche: Masculinity and the justification of meat consumption. *Psychology of Men & Masculinity, 14*(4), 363–377.

Roundtree, K. (2005). *A critical sociology of bodybuilding.* Master of Arts Thesis, University of Texas, Arlington.

Sagoe, D., Molde, H., Andreassen, C. S., Torsheim, T., & Pallesen, S. (2014). The global epidemiology of anabolic-androgenic steroid use: A meta-analysis and meta-regression analysis. *Annals of Epidemiology, 24*(5), 383–398.

Samaritans. (2012). *Men, suicide and society. Research report.* www.samaritans.org

Scambor, E., Bergmann, N., Wojnicka, K., Belghiti-Mahut, S., Hearn, J., Holter, O. G., Gärtner, M., Hrženjak, M., Scambor, C., & White, A. (2014). Men and gender equality: European insights. *Men & Masculinities, 17*, 552–577.

Seidler, V. J. (1994). *Unreasonable men: Masculinity and social theory.* London: Routledge.

Seidler, V. (2007). Masculinities, bodies, and emotional life. *Men and Masculinities, 10*, 9–21.

Shilling, C. (1993). *The body and social theory.* London: Sage.

Silverstein, L. B., Auerbach, C. F., & Levant, R. F. (2002). Contemporary fathers reconstructing masculinity: Clinical implications of gender role strain. *Professional Psychology, Research and Practice, 33*, 361–369.

Simpson, M. (1994). *Male impersonators: Men performing masculinity.* London: Cassell.

Simpson, M. (2002). Meet the metrosexual. *Salon.* Retrieved January 4, 2008, from http://dir.salon.com/story/ent/feature/2002/07/22/metrosexual/index2.html

Simpson, R. (2004). Men in non-traditional occupations: Career entry, career orientation and experience of role strain. *Gender, Work & Organization, 12*(4), 363–380.

Singleton, P., Fawkner, H.J., White, A., & Foster, S. (2009, October 8). Men's experience of cosmetic surgery: A phenomenological approach to discussion board data. *Qualitative Methods in Psychology Newsletter*, pp. 17–23.

Sloan, C. E., Gough, B., & Conner, M. T. (2015). How does masculinity impact on health? A quantitative study of masculinity and health behavior in a sample of UK men and women. *Psychology of Men & Masculinity, 16*, 206–217.

Smith, J. A., & Robertson, S. (2008). Men's health promotion: A new frontier in Australia and the UK? *Health Promotion International, 23*, 283–289.

Smith, D., Rutty, M. C., & Olrich, T. W. (2016). Muscle dysmorphia and anabolic-androgenic steroid use. In M. Hall, S. Grogan, & B. Gough (Eds.), *Chemically modified bodies: The use of substances for appearance enhancement.* Basingstoke: Palgrave.

Sparkes, A. C., & Smith, B. (2002). Sport, spinal cord injury, embodied masculinities, and the dilemmas of narrative identity. *Men & Masculinities, 4*(3), 258–285.

Stevenson, N., Jackson, P., & Brooks, K. (2000). The politics of 'new' men's lifestyle magazines. *European Journal of Cultural Studies, 3,* 366–385.

Stibbe, A. (2004). Health and the social construction of masculinity in Men's health magazine. *Men & Masculinities, 7,* 31–51.

Stice, E., Marti, N. C., Spoor, S., Presnell, K., & Shaw, H. (2008). Dissonance and healthy weight eating disorder prevention programs: Long-term effects from a randomized efficacy trial. *Journal of Consulting and Clinical Psychology, 76*(2), 329–340.

Sullivan, C. F. (2003). Gendered cybersupport: A thematic analysis of two online cancer support groups. *Journal of Health Psychology, 8*(1), 83–103.

Sullivan, C. F. (2008). Cybersupport: Empowering asthma caregivers. *Pediatric Nursing, 34*(3), 217–224.

Taylor, N. L. (2011). "Guys, he's humongous!" gender and weight-based teasing in adolescence. *Journal of Adolescent Research, 26,* 178–199.

Thompson, E. H., & Pleck, J. H. (1986). The structure of male role norms. *American Behavioral Scientist, 29,* 531–543.

Throsby, K., & Gill, R. (2004). It's different for men: Masculinity and IVF. *Men & Masculinities, 6,* 330–348.

Treadwell, H. M., & Young, A. M. W. (2012). The right US men's health report: High time to adjust priorities and attack disparities. *American Journal of Public Health, 103,* 5–6.

Valkonen, J., & Hänninen, V. (2012). Narratives of masculinity and depression. *Men & Masculinities, 16*(2), 160–180.

Walker, C., & Roberts, S. (Eds.). (2017). *Masculinity, labour and neoliberalism: Working class men in international perspective.* Basingstoke: Palgrave.

Watson, J. (2000). *Male bodies: Health, culture and identity.* Buckingham: Open University Press.

Weinland, J. A. (2009). The lived experience of informal African American male caregivers. *American Journal of Men's Health, 3*(1), 16–24.

Wetherell, M. (2012). *Affect and emotion: A new social science understanding.* London: Sage.

Wetherell, M., & Edley, N. (1999). Negotiating hegemonic masculinity: Imaginary positions and psycho-discursive practices. *Feminism & Psychology, 9*(3), 335–356.

Wetherell, M., & Edley, N. (2014). A discursive psychological framework for analyzing men and masculinities. *Psychology of Men & Masculinities,* 355–365.

Wilkins, D. (2007). The research base for male obesity: What do we know? In A. White & M. Pettifer (Eds.), *Hazardous waist: Tackling male weight problems* (pp. 3–11). Abingdon: Radcliffe Publishing.

Wilkins, D. (2010). *Untold problems: A review of the essential issues in the mental health of men and boys.* London: Men's Health Forum.

Willott, S., & Griffin, C. (1997). 'Wham, bam, am I a man?': Unemployed men talk about masculinities. *Feminism & Psychology, 7*(1), 107–128.

Wong, J., Steinfeldt, J., Hickman, S., & Speight, Q. (2010). Content analysis of the psychology of men & masculinity (2000–2008). *Psychology of Men & Masculinity, 11*, 170–182.

Wyllie, C., Platt, S., Brownlie, J., Chandler, A., Connolly, S., Evans, R., Kennelly, B., Kirtley, O., Moore, G., O'Connor, R., & Scourfield, J. (2012). *Men, suicide and society.* The Samaritans. Retrieved from: http://www.samaritans.org/sites/default/files/kcfinder/files/Men%20and%20Suicide%20Research%20Report%20210912.pdf

INDEX

© The Author(s) 2018
B. Gough, *Contemporary Masculinities*,
https://doi.org/10.1007/978-3-319-78819-7

CPSIA information can be obtained
at www.ICGtesting.com
Printed in the USA
LVHW04*1243280518
578670LV00011B/676/P

9 783319 788180